Enhancing Fertility through Functional Medicine

Enhancing Fertility through Functional Medicine: Using Nutrigenomics to Solve 'Unexplained' Infertility provides cutting-edge information and solutions to help support the worldwide rise of fertility challenges. It addresses common, yet not commonly known, root causes of oxidative stress that are at the heart of reproductive issues (and all chronic health issues). These solutions can help enhance the outcomes of assisted reproductive technologies (ART) or support women to avoid them altogether.

Enhancing Fertility through Functional Medicine: Using Nutrigenomics to Solve 'Unexplained' Infertility will show you how to improve cell health (including egg and sperm), lower inflammation, balance nervous system functioning, and optimize genetic expression, allowing the body to return to its naturally fertile state. It details information on numerous root causes of health-derailing inflammation and oxidative stress, while the appendices discuss the genetic and biochemical pathways related to these topics.

Each chapter also provides easy "Action Steps" that can be implemented immediately. Chapter topics include iron dysregulation; oxalates; mold/mycotoxins; phase 2 liver detoxification pathways; fat utilization; introductory information on genetics, epigenetics, and nutrigenomics; everything one needs to know about histamine intolerance; and how these factors adversely affect metabolic and reproductive functions.

Enhancing Fertility through Functional Medicine: Using Nutrigenomics to Solve 'Unexplained' Infertility is *the* handbook for people wanting to achieve and sustain a healthy pregnancy. It highlights lesser-known causes of fertility challenges the reader can learn how to investigate. This book also serves as a reference guide for practitioners, providing them with additional tools to add to their repertoires when other protocols have not been effective. It may also provide clarity as to *why* other protocols did not work and will enable the practitioner to custom-tailor protocols for each patient.

Endorsements

Jaclyn Down's book *Enhancing Fertility through Functional Medicine* takes a fresh and updated look at many common but lesser knows root triggers in infertility, such as important genetic variants beyond MTHFR and mold toxicity. Jaclyn draws upon her wealth of experience in this step-by-step guidebook to help you overcome fertility and achieve a healthy pregnancy and healthy baby. If you're a fertility practitioner looking for new ideas or you're struggling with fertility issues yourself and seeking answers, you'll want to check out the cutting-edge information in this book.

—Beth O'Hara, FN | Functional Naturopath | Mast
Cell Activation and Histamine Specialist
mastcell360.com
www.facebook.com/MastCell360

There is no doubt about it! We are living in a toxic environment that will cause more and more illness as time goes on. Fertility is impacted big time and perhaps will be the major issue in this decade. Jaclyn Downs has written a vital book that discusses the new genetics, the environment, illness, fertility and more. She offers sophisticated and easy solutions that work. This book is highly recommended; and in simple terms, perhaps the secret remedy to assist in sustaining our civilization!

—Stephen T. Sinatra, MD, FACC
Cardiologist and Author

After struggling with fertility for several years, it eventually felt like a disheartening guessing game trying to discover what wasn't working. It was so refreshing to finally have a resource with a span of root issues thoroughly explained followed by solutions to establish optimal fertility and an ideal biological environment to carry a baby. It brought so much clarity, understanding, and hope! Thank you, Jaclyn, for creating this beautiful guidebook.

Lauren Scruggs Kennedy
Lifestyle blogger and bestzselling author

As a practitioner in the space of treating fertility challenges for 20 years, I have found that this book provides any fertility practitioner with the tools to address the most commonly overlooked root cause fertility problems so that their patients may benefit and bring home their dream baby. This book is also a great resource for the highly motivated fertility patient who is not getting the support or answers she needs on her path to motherhood. Functional Fertility has an abundant amount of science backed information to help both patients and their practitioners discover the underlying reason(s) for fertility challenges & hormonal imbalance.

Aimee E. Raupp, Best-selling author,
acupuncturist & fertility expert

Enhancing Fertility through Functional Medicine

Using Nutrigenomics to Solve 'Unexplained' Infertility

Jaclyn Downs, MS, CHC, CD

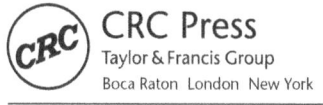

CRC Press
Taylor & Francis Group
Boca Raton London New York

CRC Press is an imprint of the
Taylor & Francis Group, an **informa** business

First edition published 2023
by CRC Press
6000 Broken Sound Parkway NW, Suite 300, Boca Raton, FL 33487–2742

and by CRC Press
4 Park Square, Milton Park, Abingdon, Oxon, OX14 4RN

CRC Press is an imprint of Taylor & Francis Group, LLC

© 2023 Taylor & Francis Group, LLC

Library of Congress Cataloging-in-Publication Data
Names: Downs, Jaclyn, author.
Title: Enhancing fertility through functional medicine : using nutrigenomics to solve 'unexplained' infertility / Jaclyn Downs.
Description: First edition. | Boca Raton : CRC Press, 2023. | Includes bibliographical references and index. | Summary: "Enhancing Fertility through Functional Medicine: Using Nutrigenomics to Solve 'Unexplained' Infertility provides cutting-edge information and solutions to help support the worldwide rise of fertility challenges. It addresses common, yet not commonly known, root-causes of oxidative stress that are at the heart of reproductive issues (and all chronic health issues). These solutions can help enhance the outcomes of Assisted Reproductive Technologies (ART) or support women to avoid them altogether. Enhancing Fertility through Functional Medicine: Using Nutrigenomics to Solve 'Unexplained' Infertility will show you how to improve cell health (including egg and sperm), lower inflammation, balance nervous system functioning, and optimize genetic expression, allowing the body to return to its naturally fertile state. It details information on numerous root causes of health-derailing inflammation and oxidative stress, while the appendices discuss the genetic and biochemical pathways related to these topics. Each chapter also provides easy "Action Steps" that can be implemented immediately. Chapter topics include iron dysregulation; oxalates; mold/mycotoxins; phase 2 liver detoxification pathways; fat utilization; introductory information on genetics, epigenetics, and nutrigenomics; everything one needs to know about histamine intolerance; and how these factors adversely affect metabolic and reproductive functions. Enhancing Fertility through Functional Medicine: Using Nutrigenomics to Solve 'Unexplained' Infertility is the handbook for people wanting to achieve and sustain a healthy pregnancy. It highlights lesser-known causes of fertility challenges the reader can learn how to investigate. This book also serves as a reference guide for practitioners, providing them with additional tools to add to their repertoires when other protocols have not been effective. It may also provide clarity as to why other protocols did not work, and will enable the practitioner to custom-tailor protocols for each patient"—Provided by publisher.
Identifiers: LCCN 2022040176 (print) | LCCN 2022040177 (ebook) | ISBN 9781032376790 (hardback) | ISBN 9781032376776 (paperback) | ISBN 9781003341369 (ebook)
Subjects: MESH: Fertility | Infertility–prevention & control | Nutrigenomics
Classification: LCC RG201 (print) | LCC RG201 (ebook) | NLM WP 565 | DDC 618.1/78–dc23/eng/20230113
LC record available at https://lccn.loc.gov/2022040176
LC ebook record available at https://lccn.loc.gov/2022040177

ISBN: 9781032376790 (hbk)
ISBN: 9781032376776 (pbk)
ISBN: 9781003341369 (ebk)

DOI: 10.1201/b23201

Typeset in Times
by Apex CoVantage, LLC

Dedication

To my father, Bill Downs, my first nutrition teacher

and my colleague, Robert Miller

and to my brilliant and inspiring daughters,
Jonen and Juno

Contents

PART 1: Introduction to Functional Fertility and Oxidative Stress

PART 2: Your 12-Week Functional Fertility Solution

Foreword

I am grateful my colleague introduced me to Jaclyn Downs. She suggested that I add her lectures to my library at Healthy Seminars, an online continuing education platform for Chinese medicine, naturopaths, chiropractors, and other professionals interested in functional and integrative medicine. As the director of Healthy Seminars, I conduct due diligence before accepting speakers to lecture. As I assessed her knowledge and experience, Jaclyn suggested I read her new book as part of my process of getting to know her professionally. Immediately upon completing her book, not only did I acknowledge that she had the academic training and clinical experience to make her an authority on infertility issues, but she had some valuable insight and information to share with those struggling with infertility.

Chinese medicine has a poetic saying when it comes to fertility: "Nourish the soil before you plant the seed." Have you ever neglected a plant to the point where the leaves turn brownish, and the plant appears slightly withered? Then by adding water, some plant fertilizer, and adjusting how much direct sunlight exposure it receives, you witness the plant regain its vigor and give off fruits and flowers. The plant always had the potential to give off fruits and flowers; however, its sub-optimal soil prevented it from reaching its peak fertility potential. You did not need to use donor roots in this case as it was the soil surrounding the roots and not the roots themselves causing the plant to wither. In this analogy, the soil is the cellular environment, and the seeds are eggs and sperm cells. Jaclyn provides us with a detailed road map on how to nourish our soil so eggs, sperm, and uterine receptivity can reach their peak fertility potential, whether trying to conceive naturally or with assisted reproductive techniques like in vitro fertilization (IVF). Jaclyn shares the same goal for those wanting to get pregnant, to conceive with more ease, and to deliver a healthy baby and healthy parent(s), too.

One of the most frustrating infertility diagnoses is unexplained infertility because no "standard" infertility testing has concluded a cause for the failure to get pregnant or maintain a pregnancy (miscarriage), so, without a known cause, there is not always an obvious treatment approach. Doctors can be challenged to suggest a specific plan because they do not know where the infertility problem lies. What if your infertility was not unexplained? What if we acted like forensic auditors and searched for what is causing embryo quality issues or implantation failure? By digging for and uncovering the root cause, we could then devise a focused approach to address the causes leading to infertility or miscarriages. Before becoming a doctor of traditional Chinese medicine, I had a career as a chartered professional accountant (CPA). I bring this auditor mindset into conducting fertility workups where my clinic provides our patients a fertility audit. We go well beyond the standard fertility workup and include a deep dive into your health by using naturopathic and functional medicine testing in addition to the standard work-up as well as the sage wisdom of Chinese medicine diagnosis in our clinic. This is why I was so happy when I received a copy of Jaclyn's book, *Enhancing Fertility through Functional Medicine: Using Nutrigenomics to Solve 'Unexplained' Infertility*. Her book delivers the reader the tests used to conduct a thorough fertility audit. Jaclyn is intentionally using quotes around the word 'unexplained' in her title as oftentimes, what is considered unexplained through the lens of conventional medicine is explainable through the lens of naturopathic, functional, and Chinese medicine.

Jaclyn offers readers some of the common areas often overlooked in the fertility assessment. She uncovers how inflammation can be one of the common causes for infertility and implantation failure and, more importantly, how to address it naturally. I often use the term "inflamm-aging" because chronic systemic inflammation causes accelerated biological aging that leads to degenerative diseases and premature fertility decline. This inflammation can be caused by poor digestive function, past trauma, the foods you eat, invisible toxins and molds in your environment, nutritional deficiencies, blood sugar issues, and stress, to name a few. She conveys loudly how oxidative stress can impair fertility, and she details some common but lesser-known factors that cause it. In her book, Jaclyn challenges the reader to search for the root cause using her road map. Her map guides us where to look, what tests to perform, and how to address the issue(s) causing infertility, implantation failure, and miscarriages. I invite you to use this book with your fertility health-care team as a resource. Reading Jaclyn's book and following her action steps at the end each chapter may be the factors that can change a diagnosis from "unexplained" to explainable to being pregnant.

Embryo quality is dependent on egg and sperm health. The embryo requires a lot of energy to divide and grow (in the fallopian tube or in the IVF lab) and to implant into the lining of the uterus, and this energy comes from the mitochondria (battery of the cell) of the egg. It gave me even more confidence in Jaclyn's thorough knowledge of reproductive health when I read her original paragraph on using low-level laser therapy (LLLT), also known as photobiomodulation, to optimize fertility by improving mitochondrial function. I am honored that she had me contribute to the section in her book on LLLT for fertility as I have observed this treatment modality as having potential and promise for addressing infertility and uterine receptivity.

It is my hope that Jaclyn's book will act as a resource for fertility practitioners and the motivated layperson trying to conceive and hoping to sustain their pregnancy. The steps in her book outline how to look for common causes as well as frequently overlooked issues that fit into the fertility landscape. This book provides bite-size actions that can be implemented immediately and/or with the support of a functional medicine or Chinese medicine practitioner.

In addition to my role at Healthy Seminars, I am also the founder and clinical director of an integrative fertility practice in Vancouver, British Columbia, Canada. I am the author of the book *Missing the Point* and the online book *The Acubalance Fertility Diet*, and I am the chair of the Integrated Fertility Symposium. I feel confident when I say Jaclyn's book will help practitioners and clients identify and address root causes of impaired fertility and help solve the infertility puzzle.

Lorne Brown DrTCM, BSc, CPA, FABORM, CHt
Chair of the Integrative Fertility Symposium
Clinical Director of Acubalance Wellness Centre (Vancouver, Canada)
President of Healthy Seminars
Author of *Missing the Point* and the online *Acubalance Fertility Diet*

Acknowledgments

Bill Downs, your love and support made me know that publishing this book was possible, and your professional experience took my book to the next level. I love you, Dad.

Charles Brommer, my husband, thank you for your endless patience, love, and support on all possible levels.

Debasis Bagchi, virtual hugs and tremendous thanks to you for introducing me to Randy Brehm.

Randy Brehm, thank you for all your guidance and for your trust in my book.

Tom Connelly, thank you for your patience in answering all my questions.

Nicole Brouse Ziegler, thank you for being my friend all these years and for the awesome cover design!!

Diane Goslin, my midwife extraordinaire, mentor, and caring friend, without you, I may never have gotten on this path.

Catherine Bonser, thank you for helping me get clarity. I look forward to continuing to work together.

Emily Givler, you are an endless well of knowledge. Thank you for sharing it.

It is with endless gratitude that I acknowledge my beta readers:

In memory of the late Dr. Stephen Sinatra, who devoted his life to improving the quality of life for others. He was an innovative pioneer and icon in integrative medicine. I will forever be grateful for his kind willingness to beta read my book and for calling me to give me his thoughtful suggestions. That was one of the highlights of writing my book!

Shivan Sarna, thank you for your time and useful input when I know you had a million other things going on.

Mackay Rippey, without you, the book wouldn't be as organized or coherent. Thank you so much for sharing your thoughts and asking the hard questions to make my content more specific.

Lauren Scruggs Kennedy, thank you for supporting my approach to fertility and for writing a review for my book.

Beth O'Hara, thank you for being a wealth of information and for your support and book review.

Ava Bird, thank you for all the time you gave to me and my book to comb over the details. I fully felt your support.

Deborah Hollinger, your heartfelt comments and suggestions are appreciated more than you know. Thank you for allowing me to reach back out to you.

Better Health Guy, Scott Forsgren, your brilliant, honest, and helpful input will forever be appreciated.

Amanda Krause, I'm so glad our paths crossed at the right time so that you were able to share your thoughts and input to help shape my book.

Monica Cox, you are a strong female force, and I am so thankful to have gotten to know you both professionally and personally. Thank you for all your encouragement and guidance!

Joy Lechner, thank you for being my cheerleader and for introducing me to Lorne Brown.

Lorne Brown, thank you for your willingness to write the foreword for this book and for your contributing words. I am excited for future collaborations.

Carly Huff Sink, thank you for your enthusiasm and support.

I'd also like to thank Dr. Joel Rosen and Aimee Raupp.

Author Biography

Jaclyn Downs is a functional nutrigenomics consultant who has a passion for fertility optimization and reproductive wellness. Through the use of functional lab testing, detailed health history, symptoms, genetics, and environmental and epigenetic influences, she works with fertility practitioners and clients to give them insight and tools to better determine root causes of reproductive challenges. Jaclyn has a bachelor of science degree in psychology from Drexel University and a master's degree in holistic nutrition. In addition to being a certified health coach, she holds a certification in genetic nutrition with the NutriGenetic Research Institute, where she is also a researcher. Jaclyn is also an author of a number of peer-reviewed published papers. She can be contacted through her website, JaclynDowns.com.

Jaclyn's other interests, hobbies, and passions include being with her husband and two awesome daughters, being outside, doing yoga, learning the banjo, and any and all things involving bicycles and roller skates.

You can contact her at Info@JaclynDowns.com.

Introduction

An infertility diagnosis delivers heavy emotions and confusing possibilities. Hundreds of articles on PubMed[1] discuss the association of infertility to depression and anxiety. But what isn't mentioned in these articles is the frustration and puzzlement that accompany alternations between hope, excitement, and despair.

Desperately wanting answers and success, someone with this diagnosis will often place their trust in a practitioner or clinic that either tries a one-size-fits-all protocol on them or treats them as just another numbered manilla file folder.

Many practitioners also experience frustration and puzzlement themselves when an infertility diagnosis is made because they want success for their patients/clients, too.

It is when the practitioner takes the time to learn the patient's *full* history, including all types of stressors, digestive functioning, physical activity levels, toxic and environmental exposures, immune system health, detailed dietary tendencies, adverse childhood events, and genetic predispositions and really *listens to* and *sees* their patients that the actual root causes can begin to be revealed.

When practitioners challenge themselves and learn to use new tools, such as genomic analysis and functional lab testing, and when they stay abreast of cutting-edge research, *then those root causes can begin to be successfully addressed.*

Optimal health can be defined as the body's ability to create and maintain an ideal biological environment; this is a drastically different premise than just the "absence of symptoms." This is especially important for women and men wanting to have babies. I wrote this book as a way to help both practitioners and their patients find and correct root causes and achieve an ideal biological environment: a healthy body primed for optimal fertility, problem-free reproduction, and healthy babies. My unique approach has led to many successful pregnancies, complete with robust, healthy, happy children! Every*body* has different needs that must be addressed for healthy fertility, and this book can be your guide to what those needs may be and how to navigate them. Whether you are personally experiencing fertility challenges or you work with patients/clients who are, this book will provide many clinical pearls and show you some very important rocks to turn over.

Part 1 of the book includes only two chapters. Chapter 1 introduces and defines what functional nutrigenomics and functional genomic fertility are, how I've created a "functional fertility" approach, and how that provides deeper insight into fertility challenges. I also describe the evolution of my approach. Chapter 2 heartily introduces oxidative stress and how this is at the root of many, if not most, fertility and reproductive challenges. I want the term "oxidative stress" to become common knowledge!

Part 2 consists of the factors that contribute to oxidative stress, broken down into 12 weeks. Each chapter in Part 2 is a different week that details a "rock to look under" that may be a root cause of fertility issues. I include information about genetics that are related to these factors, but *you will not need to know your genetics to get benefits from this book.*

This book was originally written for fertility practitioners (medical doctors, naturopaths, coaches, reproductive endocrinologists, chiropractors, acupuncturists, or any other practitioner who works with patients/clients who come to them for help with fertility). I later decided to expand to a broader audience as so many people are experiencing fertility issues, and most of them are hungry for more information than their practitioners have given them. In order to speak to both audiences, I have created appendices for the more technical, biochemical, clinical, and genetic information. Throughout the book, I state when my readers can turn to a specific appendix to gain deeper knowledge on a topic that I've mentioned.

THE LONG EVOLUTION OF MY EXPERTISE

In the first chapter, I describe how I've had an enthusiasm and hunger for learning about nutrition ever since I was a child. (My father has been in the industry since the 1980s.) Although this was something that I was interested in pursuing as a career, I put that on hold in my early 20s when I fell into birthwork and fell in love with it! I completed training to become a certified doula and also apprenticed with a very busy homebirth midwife for over five years, learning about prenatal health and natural remedies and attending over 100 births, including a few twin births and many breech births. I also became very familiar with infertility and miscarriage management.

It was also during these years that I created an on-call doula and reproductive wellness collective that gave workshops on various topics like correcting period problems, optimizing fertility, navigating the trimesters of pregnancy, and breastfeeding and cloth diapering education and tips.

When the time came for me to start a family, I experienced healthy pregnancies and gave birth to both my daughters at home, with the help of my midwife mentor. I also nursed each child for approximately three years; talk about putting my knowledge and experience into action!

Intermittently throughout my birthwork career, I also worked to advance and enhance my nutrition education. I received certification as a health coach, and I had my own wellness column in a popular local magazine for numerous years. I attended school for a master's degree in holistic nutrition before getting a job as a genomics research assistant, ultimately becoming the functional genomic nutrition consultant I am today. I still continue to attend trainings and master classes in functional nutrition and holistic health.

I have seen what has worked for fertility and what has not, and I have an understanding of *why* those things did or didn't work for each individual.

The most common and accepted way that fertility challenges are dealt with is through forcing hormones to be within certain ranges. This is not addressing the reason behind *why* the hormones are out of range or *why* the body has taken reproduction off the priority list. The human body is programmed to procreate, but it is inherently wise, too. It knows when it is *and isn't* in a safe and ideal state to procreate. Artificially manipulating the body to make a baby doesn't often end successfully because the underlying reasons have not been addressed.

My aim for this book is for my readers' overall takeaway to be that in order to get the body into a fully fertile state, one must

- Balance the limbic system, getting it out of "fight or flight" mode and into "rest, digest, repair, and reproduce" mode. This has also been called the "feed and breed" state.
- Address causes of oxidative stress.
- Get rid of things burdening the body (like toxins and dietary insults).
- Provide optimal nourishment to put the body into a fully fertile state.

And I provide action steps for each of the informational points!

Since it takes a *minimum* of 12 weeks to prepare an egg for conception (via creating an optimal environment for the egg to develop), each of the chapter topics in Part 2 of this book can be used as a guide for factors to explore each week to optimize fertility. However, I strongly recommend allowing plenty more time than 12 weeks because:

1. The lifestyle changes that I mention can take some time to implement.
2. It can take a while to replete deficient nutrient levels.
3. Toxins can take *much* longer than 12 weeks to be detoxified from the body, and it is not a "one and done" thing in this toxic world in which we live.

Because of these points, this book is not for someone who wants to skip over the foundational steps and just find a magic supplement. It is not for someone who isn't willing to put in months of prep work to get their body out of an alarm state and into a healthy reproductive state.

This book is for anyone wanting to create a healthy baby – whether that is someone experiencing fertility challenges themselves or a practitioner who wants more answers so they can help more clients have a higher success rate or even someone who may want to optimize their chances of having a healthy baby *some*day.

Reading this book and following the action steps that resonate with you *will* move you and/or your patients into a healthier state, both physically and emotionally, creating healthier eggs and sperm and allowing for an ideal environment in which to grow a baby.

This book is a great place to start at any point in your fertility journey. It will save you a tremendous amount of time, heartache, and money, as well as making for a healthier body and a healthier baby.

SIDE NOTE:

This book is a great introduction to how genetics can be used as a framework to identify root causes of oxidative stress and inflammation, the keystones for fertility challenges (and all chronic health conditions, quite frankly).

To deepen your knowledge, I offer genomic analysis consultations to both practitioners/practices and clients so that customized interventions can be made on a case-by-case basis. Consultations provide information on the top genes that each patient or client has genetic weaknesses in, information on their functions, and actionable steps on how to confirm and support those genetic weaknesses.

These consultations benefit clients by providing them with an integral piece of their infertility puzzle that other practitioners may not have been able to provide.

Practitioners greatly benefit from the consultations, which provide them with "training wheels" to be able to immediately implement genomic analysis into their practices. It allows practitioners to "learn as they go" while being able to offer this service to each patient, starting *today*. Every patient's genetic report reflects different genetic predispositions to consider, so no two consultations will be the same. This is a great way to get started if you want to incorporate genomic analysis into your practice.

Contact me at info@JaclynDowns.com to learn more about consultations.

NOTE

1 PubMed is a free resource supporting the search and retrieval of biomedical and life sciences literature with the aim of improving health – both globally and personally. The PubMed database contains more than 32 million citations and abstracts of biomedical literature. PubMed was developed and is maintained by the National Center for Biotechnology Information (NCBI) at the US National Library of Medicine (NLM), located at the National Institutes of Health (NIH).

Part 1

Introduction to Functional
Fertility and Oxidative Stress

1 What Is Functional Genomic Fertility?

I define functional genomic fertility as "Identifying and addressing root causes of reproductive imbalances through improving nutrition, detoxification ability, lifestyle, and emotional wellness, all of which support optimal genetic expression and cellular function."

Many people I know – family, friends, and clients – are experiencing reproductive challenges. Reproductive challenges often pertain to difficulty achieving pregnancy but also include miscarriages and menstrual problems of all kinds. I am writing this book to share what I have learned through experience and years of continual, cutting-edge research about the root causes of these challenges.

The subject of nutrition has always deeply resonated with me. My nutrition education began as a child as my father is a nutritional biochemist. It was through him that I learned that conventional nutritional information was *not* what made us truly healthy. Before the days of the Atkins diet rage, my father explained to me during the bagel craze of the late 1980s that excess carbs made people overweight. This went against everything that conventional nutritional articles were conveying, and nobody took him seriously at that time. During the height of the low-fat fad in the 1990s, I learned that not all fats were bad, that there were good fats and bad fats. And I think it's safe to say that I was undoubtedly the only kid in junior high school who knew what probiotics were.

I had wanted to major in nutrition when I went to college, but there were no schools in my state that taught the kind of nutrition that I was hungry to learn. I knew there was so much more to learn than the USDA's paradigm of nutrition. While there are many great registered dieticians, I didn't want to become a dietitian because I didn't want my education to be sponsored by Cargill, Sara Lee, M&M Mars, and PepsiCo, and I certainly didn't want my job to be telling people to drink low-fat milk and eat 6 to 11 servings of carbs each day. So I got a psychology degree instead.

During the pursuit of my degree at Drexel University, I learned an incredible amount about behavior, but I also was introduced to a relatively new field of study called psychoneuroimmunology. Psychoneuroimmunology focuses on the interconnectedness of our immune system, endocrine system, and central and peripheral nervous systems and how they are affected by emotional and psychological states. It explains how things like neurotransmitters and hormones can regulate immune cells, which, in turn, communicate with the nervous system. This subject resonated with me because it broadened my understanding of health far beyond just nutrition. It explained holistic health from a scientific perspective. *As you will learn in this book, chronic stressors of various types (not just mental or emotional) can make or break fertility.*

DOI: 10.1201/b23201-2

After college, I moved out to San Diego, land of sunshine and sandwiches with sprouts on them! While there, following a conversation I had with someone in which I expressed interest in doulas, she lent me a book entitled *Immaculate Deception* by Suzanne Arms. *Immaculate Deception* questions the idea that birth is dangerous and that hospital interventions improve the birthing process. I had never considered myself much of an advocate for anything except bicycling, but this book was so entirely captivating and compelling that I decided I had to become a doula and do what I could to help women have healthy, blissful, and empowering births.

I became a doula in 2002 through UCSD's Heart and Hands program and shortly thereafter became a certified birth doula. "Doula" was a very foreign word at the time, and we were few and far between. About a year later, as fate would have it, I ended up moving back to my hometown of Lancaster, Pennsylvania, to apprentice with an internationally known and highly regarded homebirth midwife. This amazing woman was very seasoned, teaching at Midwifery Today conferences all over the world on the subjects of twins, breech births, and shoulder dystocia (when the baby's shoulder gets stuck behind the mom's pubic bone during birth). During the five years that I apprenticed with her, I learned about specific herbs and remedies for fertility, pregnancy, labor, and the postpartum period. I attended well over 100 births with her but also saw hundreds of women for prenatal visits, birthing classes, and postpartum checkups. I also got to be intimately familiar with attending to miscarriages and fertility challenges. It was also during this time that I created an on-call doula service and reproductive wellness collective. As a collective of moms, lactation consultants, and fellow doulas, we gave workshops on various topics, including fertility optimization, creating birth plans, natural feminine care products, cloth diapering, postpartum self-care, and breastfeeding.

To add to my repertoire, in 2006, I took a month off birthwork to go to the Kripalu School for Yoga and Health to become a certified yoga instructor so that I could teach prenatal and postpartum yoga in my community.

1.1 MY REALIZATION

It wasn't until I apprenticed with a homebirth midwife in Pennsylvania that I first became aware of just how common impaired fertility is. In addition to realizing how common it is, I also realized that this topic is not often openly discussed. Interestingly, many of the midwife's clients were Amish and Mennonite women. The women in these communities are expected to have babies and to have them every couple of years. (No exaggeration! I have helped an Amish woman give birth to her *16th* child! And another Amish woman had three sets of twins, also among a few singletons!) This is very much expected since any method of birth control besides the fertility awareness method[1] is not allowed. Women would frequently call on this midwife for support with the miscarriage process or with difficulty conceiving. Assisted reproductive technologies like in vitro fertilization and intrauterine insemination are also not options for these women due to their religious, social, and cultural beliefs. If impaired fertility is not uncommon in the Plain Peoples' communities, which lead much slower-paced lives, it is clear that the fast-paced, high-stress lifestyles that most standard Americans lead may include even more incidences of impaired fertility.

After working with the midwife for almost five years, I decided to move to Texas to be with my boyfriend (now husband) while he was working there for about six months. The internet was fully an everyday thing by this point, and it was during this time in Texas that I enrolled in graduate school online for holistic nutrition. Over time, I spent a couple of years working towards a master's degree and also got certified as a health coach. I didn't really get my nutrition coaching business going much before I had my first child, born at home with the help of my midwife mentor.

About a year and a half into motherhood, I contacted Robert (Bob) Miller, a local naturopath, to inquire about potential employment opportunities at his practice. As it turned out, he was interested in hiring someone to be his research assistant, researching a genetic variant called MTHFR (methylenetetrahydrofolate reductase; which I will define and detail later). What began as just MTHFR quickly expanded to other genes and then entire pathways and then how the genes in those metabolic pathways interacted with other pathways and the factors that caused them to express, circling all the way back to cellular health. Compared to all the nutritional information that I had learned up until then, I was now learning at an exponential rate!

Bob took this (and ongoing) research and, using it with 23andMe's genetic raw data, created a beta test that he applied through Microsoft Excel. As the research and popularity grew, he turned it into what is now the Functional Genomic Analysis cloud-based software that (currently) analyzes over 260,000 genetic (SNPs) (info on what SNPs are is coming in the pages ahead!). This report helps practitioners identify potential weaknesses in genetic function, especially when combined with sources of inflammation, like environmental factors, that contribute to increased production of damaging free radicals or a decreased ability to detox in various liver pathways. It also helps practitioners know how to support and/or compensate for these weaknesses. As the need for researchers grew and the number of doctors and practitioners who used the software grew, Bob formed the NutriGenetic Research Institute.

In August 2017, 23andMe suddenly changed the version of the chip that was used to turn the saliva samples into our personalized raw data. The change eliminated *thousands* of SNPs that were integral to his particular genetic report. This threw all the genetic interpretation software services into a frenzy, and Bob quickly decided to design his own chip and have it analyzed through Rutgers University. This was a blessing of sorts because we (the Nutrigenetic Research Institute and the practitioners who used it) got to cherry-pick the SNPs that we wanted to include on his chip, many of which were never included in the original 23andMe chip. His genetic test kit is called Your Functional Genomics. This kit is only available for practitioners to purchase. You are able to order this kit through me. Check out the Resources section for information on ordering.[2]

What evolved, and is ever-evolving, is a dynamic, interactive software that creates a truly personalized report based on the organization and analysis of genetic information, combined with the ability to input patient/client symptom surveys and various lab test results.

To learn a little more about how a practitioner can use the software and see a visual of one of my favorite aspects of it, refer to Appendix 1A. As I mentioned in the Introduction, I offer practitioners one-to-one training consultations to review a patient's genomic report, offering them what I see to be the top genetic variants that may be causing an issue, which tests can be used to confirm if they are expressing, and suggestions on how to support those genetic weaknesses.

Throughout all this, I was not able to be on call to attend births because I had two small children and a husband in the throes of working towards an electrical engineering degree. That time was a perfect opportunity for me to marry my experience working with reproductive wellness to the functional genomics field that was (and still is) rapidly growing. I was confident that this was where I could be of utmost service for three reasons:

- Functional genomics is extremely effective in addressing root causes of impaired fertility (as well as *all kinds* of conditions).
- There was a huge lack of practitioners sharing this emerging information.
- Fertility issues are common these days.

There were plenty of doulas, nutritionists, and yoga instructors everywhere now, but not many people *at all* who shared my unique and extremely effective approach to fertility!

The current one-dimensional modus operandi for impaired fertility involves artificially forcing hormones into certain levels. *This is not getting to the root cause of why hormones are out of balance and why the body feels it's not a safe or healthy time to procreate.* The body is so innately wise and has many checks and balances to ensure proper homeostasis. What we perceive as an imbalance is often the body's attempt to compensate for or correct a deeper imbalance.

Here is the exciting news: Functional medicine and functional genomic nutrition (also referred to as "functional nutrigenomics") are emerging as extremely effective approaches to viewing health in a causative, multidimensional manner. Functional fertility, a comprehensive integrative approach, is so effective that it is going to make the current model very quickly look archaic, nonsensical, and completely *incomplete*.

This awareness is going to change everything, and here is why:

A functional approach to the body sees it as an interconnected network of systems and pathways. If something is out of balance, functional practitioners keep asking *why* until they get to the root cause of the problem. This process takes so much more than symptoms into consideration. It looks at an individual's genetics, toxic load, nutrient status, physiology, environment, lifestyle, past exposures and traumas, stress levels, metabolic functioning, and biochemistry. *Imbalances in hormones are not solely due to the endocrine system!*

My functional nutrigenomic approach to fertility largely involves making sure there is a calm, balanced limbic system, also referred to as the "feeling and reacting brain," which is a primordial part of the brain. The limbic system is an aggregation of brain structures, including the hypothalamus, that plays a role in emotions and an important role in survival. Plenty of research has linked the limbic system to things like learning, memory, motivation, hunger, and thirst but also to functions directly related to fertility, like the production of hormones that regulate the autonomic nervous system. An easy way to remember the functional role of the autonomic nervous system is to think of it as the "automatic nervous system." I mention the autonomic nervous system numerous times throughout the book, each time making the point that *if our nervous system is in a state of stress, mating ability will be the first thing to become compromised.* Importantly, today's modern agribusiness and food processing practices push the body into a state of survival panic that contributes to exhausting immunity and compromising fertility.

My approach also highlights the points that I find most important in supporting hormone, gut, and cell health (especially eggs and sperm). In fact, all the points discussed in this book improve cellular health, both directly and indirectly. I mention mitochondria (the parts of cells that are the energy generators) *dozens* of times throughout the book because mitochondria are the *only* source of energy that the egg has, and the quality of the egg is the determining factor in achieving successful pregnancy. As women age, their mitochondrial functioning decreases, in part due to various factors that I highlight in this book. I firmly believe that through improving mitochondrial functioning, we can improve egg and sperm quality (and, undoubtedly, overall health) and improve current fertility statistics.

1.2 THE STATISTICS ON INFERTILITY AND MISCARRIAGE

I would like to preface this section by saying that I personally prefer using the term "impaired fertility" because it can connote or imply a temporary state, whereas "infertility" sounds like a dead-end diagnosis with no solutions. Impaired fertility includes the hopeful ability to overcome challenges and to achieve pregnancy, whereas infertility does not, and the purpose of this book is about restoring hope.

The number of people experiencing difficulties getting pregnant and/or sustaining a pregnancy seems ever rising. The National Institutes of Health defines infertility as not being able to achieve pregnancy after one year of having regular, unprotected intercourse or after six months if the woman is older than 35. According to the NIH, studies suggest that 12–15% of couples trying to conceive are unable to conceive after one year. I want to note that that number doesn't take into account the number of women experiencing miscarriages. For couples who do get pregnant, 10–25% will end in miscarriage. That percentage increases as maternal age increases. According to the American Pregnancy Association, women from 35 to 45 years old have a 20–35% chance of miscarriage, and women over the age of 45 can have up to a 53% chance of miscarriage. Shanna H. Swan states in *Scientific American* that it is estimated that miscarriage rates are increasing by about 1% per year. Around 80% of miscarriages occur in the first trimester, with 60% of the fetuses in first-trimester miscarriages considered "chromosomally abnormal" (Calleja-Agius et al. 2012).

Unexplained infertility is diagnosed when both partners' results on fertility testing – such as semen analysis, ovulation assessment, and tubal patency – are normal. Unexplained infertility represents the single most frequent diagnosis in female infertility, with an approximate prevalence of 25–30% of all infertility cases (Brazdova 2016).

However, this should not be a burden solely placed on the woman! The CDC states that overall, one-third of infertility cases are caused by male reproductive issues, one-third by female reproductive issues, and one-third by both male and female reproductive issues or by unknown factors. That means men actually share half the burden.

Sperm health is declining, and it's happening at an alarming rate. A meta-analysis published in the journal *Human Reproduction Update* showed that sperm counts declined by 50% in just 40 years. (Hagai Levine, November-December 2017) That's more than 10% per decade! Where will that leave us in 50 more years?

1.3 ART STATISTICS

Assisted reproductive technologies (ART) include all fertility treatments in which either eggs or embryos are physically handled or manipulated.

Just like when a woman is quickly prescribed pharmaceutical birth control for painful, irregular, sporadic, or very heavy periods, medical interventions like intrauterine insemination (IUI) and in vitro fertilization (IVF) are often quickly suggested as the only solution. These interventions are very costly, averaging $10,000 to $15,000 for a single round of IVF, and they do not address why the problem is occurring in the first place. Importantly, they do not have a very high success rate. The chance of having a full-term, normal birth weight and singleton live birth per ART cycle using fresh embryos from non-donor eggs is 21.3% for women younger than 35, according to Penn Medicine's Fertility Care blog on their most recent ART statistics (2018).

All these statistics are overwhelming and can leave a couple feeling hopeless. Approaching fertility from a functional perspective can turn these statistics around because the body has an amazing ability to heal itself to achieve its ultimate inborn desire to procreate.

We need to address the foundational blocks of health and then identify and address root causes of metabolic imbalances, all of which I describe in detail in these pages. Ideally, these issues would be addressed before venturing on an ART journey, but they will still enhance overall health and fertility in any phase of your journey. In fact, according to Foresight, a British medical association for the promotion of pre-conception, IVF success rates *more than doubled* when both partners were given an optimum nutrition method of treatment and any underlying health problems were resolved (Holford 2005).

Because a functional genomic fertility approach is so personalized, tailored to each individual's genes, health history, current symptoms, and goals, the client won't ever feel like "just a number," which is often the case with the allopathic model of care. Keep in mind, the main allopathic/medical perspective is to relieve suffering. The primary medical objective is generally not to find the cause of a problem but to treat or relieve the symptoms of dysfunctions.

A common complaint some have voiced while walking through the ART process is that of "treating the condition" with a linear "boxed" protocol. Evidence is mounting that these one-size-fits-all interventions might not work or have an unacceptable failure rate because they don't address the *individual's* underlying issues. With a functional approach, root issues are addressed to set the body up for ART to be more successful in the future, *if it is even needed at all*. The goal is supporting the whole person to improve the biological terrain so the body will work optimally.

The ultimate bonus there, though, is that through addressing these fundamental issues, we create healthier children. Throughout past decades, we have experienced a steep nosedive in fertility and in children's immune, digestive, cognitive, neurological, and behavioral health. My passion and conviction are to turn this nose-dive around to help increase the health of our future.

Although I stated previously that 10–25% of all clinically recognized pregnancies will end in miscarriage, I believe the actual number is likely higher because many miscarriages occur early in pregnancy, before a woman even realizes she's pregnant. And it is not uncommon for women to experience more than one miscarriage. A woman who has had a previous miscarriage has a 25% greater chance of having another. I didn't mention *why* miscarriages can happen, so let's take a look at some potential reasons.

According to AmericanPregnancy.org, miscarriages can happen due to any number of reasons, including:

- Exposure to environmental and workplace hazards, such as high levels of radiation or toxic agents
- Hormonal irregularities (including thyroid hormone)
- Improper implantation of fertilized egg in the uterine lining
- Disorders of the immune system, including the autoimmune diseases lupus and Hashimoto's
- Nutritional deficiencies and malnutrition (either due to poor nutrient absorption or lack of proper nutrition)
- Diabetes that is not controlled

The information I present in this book is relevant to preventing miscarriage as well as promoting fertility.

The US Department of Health and Human Services states on their website that most cases of female infertility are caused by complications with ovulation and that ovulation difficulties can be caused by hormone imbalances from a variety of causes. By the end of this book, you'll know the details of how inflammatory factors like blood sugar dysregulation, toxins, and oxalate issues cause hormone imbalances; however, much of the deeper technical information is in the appendices.

Conventional medicine sees hormonal imbalance as solely the root cause of infertility but rarely questions *why* the hormones are imbalanced. Doctors will run test after test to assess hormone levels and will prescribe doses of synthetic hormones to artificially force the body to the hormonal levels that are considered optimal for conception. This one-dimensional perspective ignores the "systems biology" (i.e., holistic) approach and still leaves a lot to be desired.

In recent years, more and more doctors are testing patients for the MTHFR genetic variant and adding that as a potential root cause of impaired fertility and miscarriage. This broadening of the conventional medicine box can be a step in the right direction, but as you will learn, can be just as big a step in the wrong direction. I do not feel that it is helpful to only test for single genetic variants unless they are known pathological genes (like muscular dystrophy). As I state numerous times in this book, no gene works in isolation. Looking at the genome and interpreting genomics functionally can tell you why you may have a fertility or chronic inflammatory issue and what could be going on that allowed that condition to occur in the first place. Only testing for MTHFR won't give you the full picture.

If this is your first time encountering this term, MTHFR is a gene that makes an enzyme involved in converting folic acid (a synthetic B vitamin) into a form of folate that our bodies require. Roughly half the population has a variant in this gene, causing that conversion to work less effectively.

An important point I want to emphasize here is that just because someone has a genetic variant does not mean that it is expressing (turned on). When a gene is expressing, it means that its genetic information is being manifested, and therefore, its enzyme/protein is being made. Harmful environmental factors that create oxidative stress (defined in the next chapter) are the major driving force that negatively affects gene expression.

By now, MTHFR has become a relatively known term, although people have different levels of understanding regarding its impact on our health and fertility. Regardless of the level of someone's understanding of MTHFR, I consider it the "gateway gene" because it is oftentimes the first gene that people become aware of, and it introduces people to the concept that genes can greatly impact our health, fertility, and longevity.

I often hear people say, "I've had miscarriages because of MTHFR," or "I can't detoxify because I have MTHFR." Yes, MTHFR may have been a contributing factor, and I'm not discounting the importance of MTHFR, but that sure is a tremendous and unreasonable amount of weight to place on a single gene.

It seems everyone is jumping on the bandwagon these days, blogging and flaunting how much they know about MTHFR, and that is only feeding the hype and keeping people focused on a single gene.

Since the beginning of (wo)man, the body has had such a tremendous wisdom for knowing when to shut off mating ability. This is usually because of a threat to safety or a lack of ability to produce enough energy to grow a human within the body. I detail these reasons, right down to a cellular, biochemical level, throughout the chapters ahead.

One of my primary objectives is to very loudly emphasize that oxidative stress (and damage), which I will be defining in detail, is a primary causative factor for impaired fertility. I will go into detail on some obvious and lesser-known root causes of oxidative stress. The quick definition of oxidative stress is when there are more damaging free radicals (atoms with an unpaired electron) than there are antioxidants that neutralize them, resulting in cellular and tissue damage. My aim is to expand the conversation about oxidative stress and make it a commonly recognized and better understood term. I want to let the world know how *profoundly* oxidative stress impacts inflammation (which is the common denominator in all chronic conditions) and, therefore, fertility. Most people vastly underestimate the amount of damage that oxidative stress can create!

There are many genes in numerous pathways that create and modulate oxidative stress levels. Because of this fact, I will be conveying why MTHFR is but one piece of a very large puzzle, and it is not the first genetic variant we should address when dealing with impaired fertility or any health concerns for that matter (and why). There are many other genes, enzymes, and cofactors that come into play that warrant discussion. And there are more pathways to bring into the fertility equation besides just methylation. Because oxidative stress is a primary component of impaired fertility, I wanted to share why this is and also detail some cutting-edge information on the root causes of inflammation. Upon learning this information, you will have the knowledge to possibly change the trajectory of your fertility journey and, ideally, complete it with a blissful pregnancy, positive birth experience with minimal intervention, and a robust baby with high potential.

Just as no gene works in isolation, there's no "magic pill" that will create optimal fertility. Taking a specific product or eating a "fertility-boosting" food is like adding one mineral to greatly depleted soil. There are just too many factors at play these days, working against our health and fertility.

Just as farmers and gardeners prepare the soil in which they will sow and grow their seeds, we must take care to prepare our bodies (physically and emotionally) to optimize growth potential when creating another beautifully complex human. As you will learn, this can impact the health and fertility potential of future generations beyond our direct offspring.

We are holistic, energetic, and spiritual beings, and everything is connected to everything else. Numerous things affect our metabolism, our ability to produce hormones, our neurotransmitter interconnectivity and balance, and our ability to ovulate and menstruate regularly. So, of course, there is no "one size fits all" remedy.

Unlike simpler, slower, pre-industrial times, we now have to go out of our way not to be infertile, toxic, nutrient depleted, depressed, and/or anxious. Our existence is truly becoming, once again, "survival of the fittest." However, "fittest" now has come to mean those who are vigilantly educating themselves and advocating for their own health and that of their potential offspring.

Unfortunately, that has not yet become the norm. Most people spend more time preparing their babies' nurseries than they do preparing their bodies to grow a human being! This is true for both the mother and the father. Most women don't think about optimizing their bodies until either they become pregnant or have become disappointed in trying to achieve or sustain a pregnancy. And most men don't consider fertility optimization at all! Tons of papers have been published that reveal how much of an influence the health of the male and sperm are on the whole process.

The good news is, with the ever-growing knowledge, education, discoveries, tools, and options we have available to us, we can reverse and restore our bodies from deficiencies, toxic burden, inflammation, and oxidative stress, thereby optimizing fertility in both men and women. In fact, almost all the information covered in this book can be applied to optimizing male fertility as well as female fertility.

Your body's top priority is healthy survival. It must feel confident that you are healthy and robust enough to endure the demands of sharing it with a growing fetus, as well as the arduous task of giving birth.

The answer to the question of "What creates fertility?" is a body that is able to have resilience from stressors. A body that is lacking, toxic, or worn down (by oxidative stress, poor thyroid and/or adrenal function, impaired energy production, food intolerances, viruses, bacterial or fungal overgrowth, etc.) inherently knows it is not a good time to create offspring. Forcing your body into pregnancy makes for a less than ideal situation. *The wise path is to get the body calm, nourished, and detoxified first, then the body will feel that it has a safe, healthy house in which to grow a healthy, beautiful being.*

This book is a practical handbook for fertility practitioners and their clients to introduce new concepts, genetics, and cutting-edge information on fertility. It is going to offer you new "rocks to look under," ones that reveal root causes of inflammation and imbalance on a bio-individual basis. It will provide you with some new and very sharp tools to add to your toolbox.

As you can see, there's so much more to impaired fertility than a variant in a single gene, imbalanced hormone levels, or fixing them with a single magic nutrient.

1.4 WHAT EXACTLY IS A HORMONE, ANYWAY?

Before we get too far along, I should define what a hormone actually is. A hormone is a protein (made up of amino acids) that is produced by cells and transported via the blood to cells and organs on which it has a regulatory effect. In other words, it is a chemical messenger that makes things happen or stops them from happening. Hormones control a huge and vital range of things in addition to sexual reproduction, like growth, control of metabolic processes, and mood/mental conditions. Instead of attempting to change the message that has been sent (by way of artificial hormones), as many doctors often do with impaired fertility, *we should ask why that is the message being sent in the first place!*

1.5 A WORD ON ASSISTED REPRODUCTIVE TECHNOLOGIES IN RELATION TO HORMONES

A rising number of people are born via in vitro fertilization. Many babies born via conventional medical ART treatments are special needs/high needs children. A 'grand theme review' in *Human Reproduction Update* poses the question of why this is, whether it is due to subfertility factors of the parents or the ART treatments themselves (Berntsen et al. 2019). In fact, higher percentages of miscarriage, preeclampsia, placenta previa, gestational diabetes, premature births, low average birth weights, perinatal mortality, cerebral palsy, and congenital defects are the new issues concerning disorders that accompany ART (Strömberg et al. 2002). Additionally, children born as a result of assisted reproductive technology were shown to be twice as likely to have autism than those born without reproductive assistance, according to study findings in the *American Journal of Public Health* (Fountain et al. 2015).

Even though we've made incredible strides in sperm and egg handling and culture conditions, the success rates of ART procedures have not. A review article published by the Cleveland Clinic entitled *Oxidative Stress and Its Role in Female Infertility and Assisted Reproduction: Clinical Implications* states that suboptimal oocytes and embryo quality are among the many reasons contributing to poor pregnancy rates after IVF/ICSI. As our understanding of the metabolism of gametes (i.e., an organism's reproductive cells) and embryos has increased over recent years, we have come to learn that oxidative stress negatively impacts human embryos and development. (Ashok 2009) We need healthy eggs and sperm to make healthy babies!

Forcing hormones to specific levels may trick the body into making a baby, but if the mother's health is out of balance from things like nutrient deficiencies, for example, she passes that on to her baby. How can the baby get enough if the mom doesn't have enough to give? You can't pour from an empty cup.

And if the mom has cortisol dysregulation, you better believe the baby will, too (Duthie and Reynolds 2013).

The limbic system is among the oldest parts of the brain, and it determines whether or not the body is in a safe state to procreate.

The limbic system regulates the autonomic nervous system and the endocrine system, which haven't evolved much over the past *thousands* of years. When we experience stress, the body doesn't really differentiate between causes of stress (physical, emotional, oxidative, environmental); it just responds the way it always has, as if a predator were chasing us. Many of us are constantly in a stressful state, with no reprieve.

In those more primal times, when we had stress, it was usually due to an encounter with a predator. When we saw that predator charging our way, our autonomic nervous system flipped the "rest, digest, repair, reproduce" switch (technically called the parasympathetic nervous system) to the "fight, freeze, or flight" switch (sympathetic nervous system). This started calling on cortisol, a primary stress hormone, to help us survive.

Cortisol helps move blood from your intestines, etc. to your arms and legs so you can defend yourself or move the heck out of harm's way. When a predator is chasing you, your body is using all its resources to deal with the stressor. It knows that now is not a safe time to make or grow a baby, so it shifts from converting cholesterol to pregnenolone (a precursor to stress and reproductive hormones) to converting cholesterol to cortisol to deal with the situation until the stressor has stopped. The reason the body shuts down reproductive hormones to deal with perceived danger is because it knows not to make a baby when danger is close *and* because using energy for reproductive health isn't essential to continue being alive; dealing with the stressor is. It makes sense, right?

Historically, what generally happened was that we started running from the predator, burned through some cortisol, got away from the danger, and then returned to homeostasis; the body is able to move back from the sympathetic "fight or flight" mode into the parasympathetic "rest, digest, repair, reproduce" mode (also called the "feed and breed" state) and replenish our cortisol stores.

For most people in Western industrialized societies in the 21st century, instead of getting chased by a predator, our stressors commonly involve things like schedules, jobs, toxins, and inflammatory foods that burden our bodies. Not to mention the added stress that trying to conceive can place on a couple! Whatever the cause of the stress, our bodies still react to it the same way that they always have.

As I've stated, using conventional allopathic ART to force the hormones to "optimal" levels isn't getting to the root of the problem of *why* the hormones are imbalanced in the first place. *In many cases, impaired fertility may be the body's innate protective mechanism preventing it from putting a pregnant mom or her baby in a primally perceived dangerous situation.* It is my job and life's passion, and now the mission of this book, to help practitioners, their clients, and consumers wanting more information to decipher what stressors (direct, indirect, environmental, genetic, etc.) could be causing imbalances.

For most of us, that predator ("daily life") rarely stops chasing us unless we give conscious thought and mindful action to mitigating intense stress and creating functional balance and nourishment.

Some women are lucky enough to easily get pregnant. But it is not uncommon for these women to have what are considered "high-risk" pregnancies and various complications or just to feel downright miserable and hate being pregnant (which, logically, isn't supposed to be, based on the fact that procreation is designed to be desirable). Additionally, the birthing process has become a dangerous act for many women, having to give birth early due to complications or spontaneous preterm labor; and the babies and children who result? A rising epidemic of allergies, neurological disorders, developmental and learning disorders, behavioral problems, autoimmune diseases, skin and respiratory issues, and birth defects is occurring.

It is not supposed to be this way, just as I know that sex is not supposed to be painful or unpleasant. (Be sure to read the chapter on oxalates if sex is physically painful for you.) Biologically, sex is supposed to be pleasant to ensure the propagation of our species, and periods aren't supposed to cause vomiting or being "laid up" from pain. Periods are supposed to be regular and uneventful and, in some circles, even celebrated. PMS and problematic or irregular periods are symptoms that the body is experiencing hormonal imbalance, toxin overload, or nutrient deficiencies and can be a major sign of potential problems getting pregnant or sustaining a pregnancy.

Luckily, the body is extraordinary at rebalancing itself, if we just create the proper biological environment for it to do so. In the pages ahead, I'm going to give you many tips and strategies to help you create that ideal environment.

Remember that studies have shown that 12 weeks is the *minimum* amount of time needed to optimize the health of the maturing egg and to balance hormones, the cornerstones of fertility. This book will help you optimize the environment in which that egg is matured. We want to create a nourished, toxin-free, inflammation-free environment so that the egg can reach its full potential! To optimize the chance of fertilization, implantation, and viability of a pregnancy, it is best to start the 12 week functional fertility solution as far in advance as possible! Give your eggs (and sperm) the advantage of a longer head start!

NOTES

1 Also referred to as natural family planning, this method involves keeping track of your monthly cycle and ovulation based on body temperature, charting, and cervical fluid consistency. This method is a great way to get you more in tune with your body, as well as for both achieving and preventing pregnancy (depending on what your goal is). There are great books written on this topic, my favorite being *Garden of Fertility* by Katie Singer.
2 I make no money in referencing this test; I just think it is a great resource that is constantly striving to be at the forefront of genetic analysis.

REFERENCES

Ashok, Agarwal, Sajal Gupta, Neena Malhotra, and Dipika Sharma. 2009. "Oxidative stress and its role in female infertility and assisted reproduction: clinical implications." *International Journal of Fertility and Sterility* 2, no. 4, 147–164.

Berntsen, Sine, Viveca Söderström-Anttila, Ulla-Britt Wennerholm, Hannele Laivuori, Anne Loft, Nan B. Oldereid, Liv Bente Romundstad, Christina Bergh, and Anja Pinborg. 2019. "The health of children conceived by ART: 'The chicken or the egg?.'" *Human Reproduction Update* 25, no. 2, 137–158.

Brazdova, Andrea, Helene Senechal, Gabriel Peltre, and Pascal Poncet. 2016. "Immune aspects of female infertility." *International Journal of Fertility & Sterility* 10.

Calleja-Agius, Jean, Eric Jauniaux, and Shanthi Muttukrishna. 2012. "Inflammatory cytokines in maternal circulation and placenta of chromosomally abnormal first trimester miscarriages." *Clinical and Developmental Immunology* 2012.

Duthie, Leanne, and Rebecca M. Reynolds. 2013. "Changes in the maternal hypothalamic-pituitary-adrenal axis in pregnancy and postpartum: influences on maternal and fetal outcomes." *Neuroendocrinology* 98, no. 2, 106–115.

Fountain, Christine, Yujia Zhang, Dmitry M. Kissin, Laura A. Schieve, Denise J. Jamieson, Catherine Rice, and Peter Bearman. 2015. "Association between assisted reproductive technology conception and autism in California." *American Journal of Public Health* 105, no. 5, 963–971.

Hagai, Levine, Niels Jørgensen, Anderson Martino-Andrade, Jaime Mendiola, Dan Weksler-Derri, Irina Mindlis, Rachel Pinotti, and Shanna H. Swan. 2017. "Temporal trends in sperm count: a systematic review and meta-regression analysis." *Human Reproduction Update* 23, no. 6, 646–659.

Holford, P. 2005. *The New Optimum Nutrition Bible*. Random House Digital.

Strömberg, Bo, Gisela Dahlquist, A. F. O. K. M. Ericson, Orvar Finnström, Max Köster, and Karin Stjernqvist. 2002. "Neurological sequelae in children born after in-vitro fertilisation: a population-based study." *The Lancet* 359, no. 9305, 461–465.

2 Oxidative Stress and Inflammation as Major Root Causes of Reproductive Issues

It really drives me bananas that there are literally *thousands* of journal papers that link inflammation to impaired fertility, but everyone seems more concerned with artificially forcing the body into "balance" with synthetic hormones or a magic pill or supplement. And just giving an anti-inflammatory like Metformin isn't getting to the root cause of the inflammation. Incidentally, recent research has linked Metformin to birth defects in offspring when taken by men in the three months prior to conception! (Wensink et al. 2022). This is like a car's check engine light being on, and rather than finding out *why* it is on, just taking the bulb out so that it is no longer illuminated.

As you can see, we've got to get to the root cause of the inflammation!

2.1 INFLAMMATION AS A CAUSE AND RESULT OF OXIDATIVE STRESS

Inflammation causes the production of free radicals, and an abundance of free radicals causes oxidative stress, which causes inflammation . . . a vicious cycle. Inflammation and oxidative stress are so intertwined that there are scholarly articles stating that one causes the other and vice versa.

Inflammation is supposed to be inherently a positive thing. Our bodies create inflammation as a response to protect themselves! Our bodies are designed to create it in response to injury, pain, or acute illness that usually lasts no longer than a few days. Acute inflammation is observable as swelling, pain, warmth, and/or redness.

The reason inflammation gets a bad rap these days is because it has become chronic. Chronic, low-grade, systemic inflammation is so insidious that it silently and slowly damages the body and causes fertility issues (and a whole host of chronic illnesses). The good news is that we can prevent chronic inflammation through diet, lifestyle, and proper detoxification.

Free radicals aren't always the bad guys either; our bodies make free radicals to fight off pathogens. It is only when they become excessive of what can be neutralized and cause oxidative stress that this becomes a problem, causing damage to cells and tissues.

To learn the scientific explanation of oxidative stress and antioxidants, as well as the top 3 primary antioxidants produced by our bodies, refer to Appendix 2A.

DOI: 10.1201/b23201-3

Free radicals are created as part of a normal byproduct of energy production, but some other causes are:

- Emotional/mental stress
- Environmental toxins such as pollution, radiation, cigarette smoke, and pesticides/herbicides
- Nutrient deficiencies
- Alcohol
- Sugar
- Refined oils
- Toxic chemicals and drugs (OTC and Rx)
- Radiation
- Many cleaning products
- Many body care products
- Infection by bacteria, parasites, and viruses
- Endocrine disrupting chemicals (xenoestrogens, BPA)
- Heavy metal toxicity
- Yeast and fungal overgrowth
- Hormonal imbalances
- A diet that includes a large percentage of processed food that is laden with chemicals and toxins like pesticides, herbicides, texturizers, flavor enhancers, preservatives, stabilizers, dyes, bleaches, etc., just to name a few.

Oxidative stress damages cells – both the information they carry and the cellular structure, permanently impairing their function. Note that in addition to pathogens, toxins, and deficiencies, oxidative stress often occurs from physical stress, mental/emotional stress, and environmental stressors.

2.2 HOW INFLAMMATION AFFECTS FERTILITY

Inflammation is associated with hormonal imbalances, autoimmunity, anatomic abnormalities (Weiss et al. 2009), intrauterine growth restriction (IUGR), preeclampsia, and a vast array of other pathologies, large and small.

Systemic inflammation sends signals to the brain, which holler to the eggs, ovaries, and testes that it's not a good time to conceive. Inflammation causes cortisol to rise in an attempt to "put out the fire." Having chronically elevated cortisol dampens production of DHEA, which is the major precursor to testosterone and estrogen, and can lower production of sperm and egg quality. I will be talking a lot about elevated cortisol in this book!

An excess of highly reactive free radicals, called reactive oxygen species (ROS) and reactive nitrogen species (RNS), results in oxidative stress, which indiscriminately can affect the functionality of all parts of the cell. Oocyte (female egg) quality is greatly affected by oxidative stress. Since oocytes provide RNA, proteins, and cellular machinery for the early zygote, oocyte quality predicts embryo quality and implantation rates (Twight 2013).

While there are literally tens of thousands of scholarly papers on the topic of oxidative stress and fertility, a 2017 journal article titled *The Role of Oxidative Stress in Female Infertility and In Vitro Fertilization* stated the following:

> Recent studies found that oxidative stress may damage the oocytes and may impair their fertilization capacity. Oxidative stress may also lead to embryo fragmentation and formation of numerous developmental abnormalities, and is regarded to be one of the important reasons of spontaneous and recurrent miscarriage. Moreover, overproduction of reactive oxygen species has a significant impact on the success of in vitro fertilization (IVF).
>
> (Wojsiat et al. 2017)

Since toxins impair a cell's ability to use oxygen and create oxidative stress that damages cells (reproductive cells are very vulnerable), even common chemicals used in body care products and in the home and workplace can cause infertility, miscarriage, and birth defects (I discuss toxins in Chapter 12). These toxins can begin to impact the body *years* before a woman would even consider wanting children. What you put into and on your body and what you put your body through *years* before getting pregnant can affect your ability to get pregnant and have healthy children, especially if you have genetic predispositions to less-than-optimal antioxidant production and/or detoxification.

There are many types of free radicals, like reactive oxygen species (ROS), also called oxygen free radicals, which I mention numerous times in this book. Other types of free radicals are reactive nitrogen species (RNS), lipid peroxides, environmentally derived free radicals, and endogenously produced [made by the body] free radicals that are generated as a byproduct of cellular metabolism. They really mess with fertility (and all other aspects of health) on a cellular level. Just know that if not kept in check, they damage DNA, oxidize important molecules in the body so they can't properly do their jobs, and can hinder many processes in the body, such as making cellular energy, known as adenosine triphosphate (ATP).

The following is just one quote from one of *many* studies and review articles on the topic of oxidative stress and fertility consequences. This one discusses free radicals (ROS) that damage cell structure and genomic material, affecting eggs, sperm, and embryos in endometriosis patients.

> ROS impedes embryo development and causes embryotoxicity and teratogenesis [creation of a malformed or deformed baby].
>
> (Máté et al. 2018)

Wrap your brain around this fact so it can blow your mind: A female baby is born with all the eggs she will ever have in her life. In fact, when a female fetus is four months gestational age, she has all the eggs she will ever have in her life; thus, the mother is carrying the seed of her grandchild within her own body! *Half your DNA was inside your mother before she was even born!!* So if you can conceive the potential possibility of ever having children, it is important to protect your precious and limited eggs, especially in these modern times when we are inundated by toxic chemicals in our environment and the food and products we purchase.

Men, on the other hand, have a bit more time to get their acts together. The sperm that a man would ejaculate today was produced roughly 70 days ago. Considering that up to 50% of a couple's infertility is due to the male, preconception optimization, especially on the man's part, can greatly enhance a couple's chance of successfully conceiving. Fertility optimization is not just a woman's job.

In the upcoming chapters, I'm going to highlight a few lesser-known but extremely prevalent causes of inflammation. To add to that, I'm going to provide you with some other common causes of inflammation and actionable ways to navigate them.

As I stated earlier, stress of all kinds impairs cellular oxygen utilization and causes oxidative damage. Let's dive a little deeper into the things that cause oxidative stress.

The lesser-known causes I'm going to highlight are:

1. Iron and copper dysregulation
2. Oxalate sensitivity
3. Poor dietary fat utilization
4. Blood sugar dysregulation
5. Mold exposure
6. Impairments in antioxidant and detoxification ability
7. Histamine intolerance

To measure some of these causes, there is a phenomenal test that reveals an incredible amount of information called a urine organic acid test (OAT). This test is a snapshot of what is currently happening metabolically in the body. It measures metabolites (organic acids) that are the byproduct/result of the body's metabolism. The OAT that the Great Plains Laboratory provides (see resources section for laboratory info) has over 70 markers for things like ability to properly use fats; mitochondrial energy production; yeast, fungal, and bacterial overgrowth; and oxalates. As you will see, I mention the benefits of this test more than a few times in this book. I want to state that I do not have any financial relationship or affiliation with Great Plains Laboratory. I just think they are "what's up" in the realm of functional lab testing, and many functional medicine practitioners consider it the leading standard!

Refer to Appendix 2B for more information on interpreting OAT results and measuring oxidative stress. I want to mention here that I am extremely well versed in the interpretation of the urine organic acids test, far beyond what is stated in the interpretation that comes with the test results. I have researched and studied each marker, and this test has been a common topic of discussion in the functional medicine circles I associate with. I am available for one-to-one consultations to interpret your or your patients' organic acid test results, in addition to consults for genomic interpretations.

I think it would be a good idea to get an OAT done before getting started so you can see what your baseline of health is before starting the 12-Week Functional Fertility Solution. Then you can do follow-up testing at the end of the 12 weeks to see how much your metabolic markers have improved. The next 12 weeks will greatly optimize your health, the health of your eggs (and sperm as well!), get your hormones balanced, and turn off the inflammatory alarm that affects your mating ability.

REFERENCES

Máté, Gábor, Lori R. Bernstein, and Attila L. Török. 2018. "Endometriosis is a cause of infertility. Does reactive oxygen damage to gametes and embryos play a key role in the pathogenesis of infertility caused by endometriosis?" *Frontiers in Endocrinology* 9, 725.

Twight, John. 2013. *Preconception nutrition and the microenvironment of the human oocyte: Proteomic and epidemiologic studies on IVF/ICSI treatment outcomes.* Erasmus University Rotterdam.

Weiss, Gerson, Laura T. Goldsmith, Robert N. Taylor, Dominique Bellet, and Hugh S. Taylor. 2009. "Inflammation in reproductive disorders." *Reproductive Sciences* 16, no. 2, 216–229.

Wensink, Maarten J., Ying Lu, Lu Tian, Gary M. Shaw, Silvia Rizzi, Tina Kold Jensen, Elisabeth R. Mathiesen, Niels E. Skakkebæk, Rune Lindahl-Jacobsen, and Michael L. Eisenberg. 2022. "Preconception antidiabetic drugs in men and birth defects in offspring: a nationwide cohort study." *Annals of Internal Medicine* 175, no. 5, 665–673.

Wojsiat, Joanna, Jerzy Korczyński, Marta Borowiecka, and Żbikowska Halina Małgorzata. 2017. "The contribution of oxidative stress to female infertility and in vitro fertilization." *Advances in Hygiene and Experimental Medicine* 71.

Part 2

*Your 12-Week Functional
Fertility Solution*

3 Improving Sleep Quality as a Solid Foundation for Fertility

Before we begin, we must lay an important foundation; upgrade your sleeping habits! All the things I mention in this book won't be as effective if your sleep quality is crummy. Because it is so integral for your physical and emotional health, your sleep quality will absolutely affect your ability to conceive. You must make quality sleep a priority.

When we sleep, our immune system surveys the body and turns up the dial on detoxification. Sleep is so important to our health that approximately one-third of each day is taken up by it. It is crucial for not only our physical and mental health, but also our willingness and ability to accomplish all the daily tasks required and desired of us. So why are so many people not getting enough?

For thousands of years, we slept in darkness. Even if we slept near a campfire, there was an obvious day/night cycle with which our bodies harmonized.

Today, we rarely sleep in complete darkness. We have light from our clocks, screens, nightlights, and other electronic devices in our bedrooms, as well as streetlights and lights outside our homes, illuminating our bedrooms and disrupting our circadian rhythms.

Blue light exposure from screens before bed can greatly affect your sleep and potentially cause disease, according to the Harvard Health Letter. While light of any kind can suppress the secretion of melatonin and disrupt a person's circadian rhythm, blue light at night has the worst effect.

Our circadian rhythm, also referred to as our "sleep/wake cycle," does more than regulate our sleep. It influences our immune system, mental health, and cognitive function, as well as our metabolism, cell regeneration, and eating habits. Two other things it also influences/regulates are our body temperatures and hormonal regulation, and as you may know, waking basal body temperature is a marker for hormonal health and fertility. Our circadian rhythm is our body's master clock that controls biochemical processes on a 24-hour cycle. Because it operates in concert with every organ and gland, it regulates many aspects of our physiology and behavior. When it is out of whack, all the functions that it regulates are affected.

Melatonin is a naturally occurring hormone in the body that affects sleep and circadian rhythm, as well as immunity and reproduction (Gao et al. 2019). In addition to being a hormone, melatonin is also a potent antioxidant and anti-inflammatory. Melatonin protects mitochondria from oxidative damage. If mitochondria are damaged, our cells will not create energy. The body inherently knows that it is not an ideal time to try to grow a human being if it doesn't have ample energy-producing ability. But

DOI: 10.1201/b23201-5

before considering supplementing with this powerful hormone, I highly advise that you have a discussion with your health practitioner first.

Disruptions in circadian rhythm can alter blood sugar regulation. Studies show a link between circadian rhythm disruption and diabetes (Hudec et al. 2020), obesity, and metabolic syndrome (Zimmet et al. 2019). In Chapter 15, I discuss how blood sugar dysregulation affects fertility. Circadian rhythm balance is an important factor for healthy blood sugar regulation and, therefore, fertility.

ACTION STEPS

Here are some tips to help improve sleep and dial in your circadian rhythm.

- Get your sleep hygiene on. Go to bed around the same time most nights. Sleep in as dark a room as possible; otherwise, use some sort of sleep mask. If you must use any sort of light, like a night-light or a digital alarm clock, red light is the least disruptive to circadian rhythm and melatonin production.
- Sleep on the best bed you can afford to invest in.[1] You spend about a third of your 24-hour day in bed. Do not sleep on a toxic bed! Many memory foam beds are made with toxic industrial chemicals like petroleum-based polyurethane, formaldehyde, and benzene. Most beds use chemical flame retardants, which are toxic as well.
- Consider that metal coils in your mattress may act like antennas for elec-tromagnetic frequencies, especially if you are someone who charges your phone on your nightstand all night long. Since there are currently no pub-lished studies on this that I am aware of, even though there are articles writ-ten by scientists on this topic, I prefer to err on the side of caution. I also prefer to charge my phone in the evening before I head to bed. I then put it in airplane mode, which doesn't use much battery power, so it's still fresh in the morning. If you're not completely sold on this, consider it a "might help, can't hurt" point that needs further research.
- Take magnesium. This mighty mineral is relaxing to the body, and taking it at bedtime can help with sleep. It also can help with constipation, blood sugar regulation, healthy blood pressure, activation of ATP, and so many more things!
- No screens at least an hour before bed. If you feel the desire to do so, I rec-ommend blue light–blocking glasses and/or switching your phone to "night-time" mode, in which the blue light filters out so your screen has a softer glow. There are apps and free software programs you can download, like f.lux, that dial down the blue light on your computer screen as the evening progresses, based on your location.
- Get outside and have the sun's rays kiss your eyeballs when the sun is low on the horizon in the morning, at midday, and in the evening. I discuss this further in the next section, but think about it: For most of human history, we lived and worked outside, rising with the sun. It's only in the recent history of man that we have shelter and artificial light. This is also a great way to

get outside for a walk or spend some time in the garden. Try to get your light exposure without any sort of lenses over your eyes so that the full spectrum of rays can be absorbed.

Changing and/or optimizing your light-dark cycles can speed up, slow down, or reset biological clocks as well as circadian rhythms. Following these tips will not only help you have a more restful sleep but also benefit your health on numerous levels.

NOTE

1 I am not a blogger, but when I needed a real bed in a bad way when I was pregnant, I neurotically researched for over two weeks before deciding on one and then wrote about the whole experience, complete with which bed I chose and why (www.jaclyndowns.com/blog/2015/11/28/my-bed-the-most-satisfying-purchase-i-ever-made). And seven years later, it's *still* the most satisfying purchase I ever made!

REFERENCES

Gao, Juan, Han-Qiao Liu, Yan Wang, Ya-Li Shang, and Fang Hu. 2019. "Effects of psychological care in patients with endometriosis: a systematic review protocol." *Medicine* 98, no. 10.

Hudec, Michael, Pavlina Dankova, Roman Solc, Nardjas Bettazova, and Marie Cerna. 2020. "Epigenetic regulation of circadian rhythm and its possible role in diabetes mellitus." *International Journal of Molecular Sciences* 21, no. 8, 3005.

Zimmet, P., K. G. M. M. Alberti, N. Stern, C. Bilu, A. El-Osta, H. Einat, and N. Kronfeld-Schor. 2019. "The circadian syndrome: is the metabolic syndrome and much more!" *Journal of Internal Medicine* 286, no. 2, 181–191.

4 Get Salivary Genetic Testing Done That Goes above and beyond Just MTHFR and Methylation

As I've previously discussed, functional nutrigenomics looks at patterns of inflammation, detoxification pathways, cellular and mitochondrial health, fat utilization (needed to make hormones, among numerous other processes), and so much more beyond just MTHFR or methylation. Problems with any number of these factors can impact our baseline of health and the quality of our reproduction, including eggs and sperm, which can greatly affect the ability to conceive, create, and sustain a healthy embryo.

Through genomic interpretation, functional lab testing, and an in-depth case history/intake, functional genomics[1] can help reveal a great amount of information about why someone is having trouble conceiving or carrying to term and effectively personalize the care that a practitioner gives a client. I want to be clear that it is not diagnostic! Knowing your genomic profile helps shine a light on various factors that can reveal or are associated with root causes of reproductive issues (or any chronic issues).

Genomic interpretation provides predictive information that can help determine why previous treatments (including ART procedures) may have been unsuccessful and what a better-targeted treatment may be. Working with a knowledgeable practitioner can help connect the dots between physiological strengths and genetic weaknesses and help people understand their physiology, perhaps more than anyone has ever helped them before. In addition to working with my own clients, I do offer consultations with practitioners to review their clients'/patients' genetic reports.

I want to be clear that knowing someone's genetics only helps provide a clear framework. It doesn't give us the whole picture but helps us contextualize information and see how everything else fits together once we have that genetic framework, especially when it is combined with lab testing to see what might be expressing. We can't know that by just looking at the genetics as they are not static, and there are many factors upstream and downstream that must be considered, just as environment and stress must be.

DOI: 10.1201/b23201-6

4.1 FIRST, WHAT IS A GENE?

A gene is a segment of DNA that contains all the information needed to encode for one protein. I remember learning in high school (and can still hear the class reciting all together in a bored, monotone way), "Amino acids are the building blocks of proteins." I didn't realize at the time that proteins make up *way* more than just muscle and tissue! They are also neurotransmitters, hormones, and all sorts of enzymes that make stuff happen in the body. Just like in Scrabble, where you can use letters to create words and then disassemble and reassemble them to make new words, amino acids can assemble and reassemble to make all sorts of proteins. If someone has poor protein digestion from a less-than-optimal gut (from things like infections, stress, toxins, food sensitivities, inadequate stomach acid, etc.), they may not break down protein effectively and, therefore, may lack enough amino acids to reassemble into other proteins, causing mood disorders, hormonal imbalance, and a whole host of other issues.

There are many genetic polymorphisms (i.e., the presence of genetic variations within a population) that can affect fertility. However, just because someone has a particular variant (i.e., allele) that is known to be problematic doesn't mean that it is doomed to express. That's where diet and lifestyle come into play. Research shows that 80–90% of what determines whether a "bad" genetic variant will be expressed are epigenetic factors such as stress, toxins, and nutrient deficiencies.

You may be surprised to learn that MTHFR is one of the last genes I address. Addressing this first can actually worsen inflammation, which I'll be discussing in detail. In fact, I almost subtitled this book "Why MTHFR Is a Gateway Gene."

Only looking at MTHFR is like thinking that you know what a complex puzzle looks like based on two pieces.

Or, for a more relevant analogy, this is MTHFR (Figure 4.1):

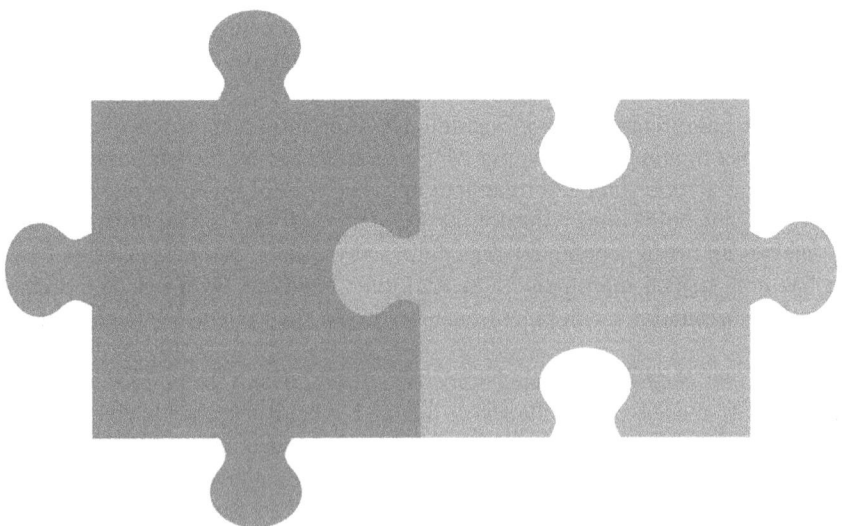

FIGURE 4.1 MTHFR is one gene in the methylation pathway that is interconnected with numerous other pathways and genes.

And these are the genetic biochemical pathways in the body (Figure 4.2):

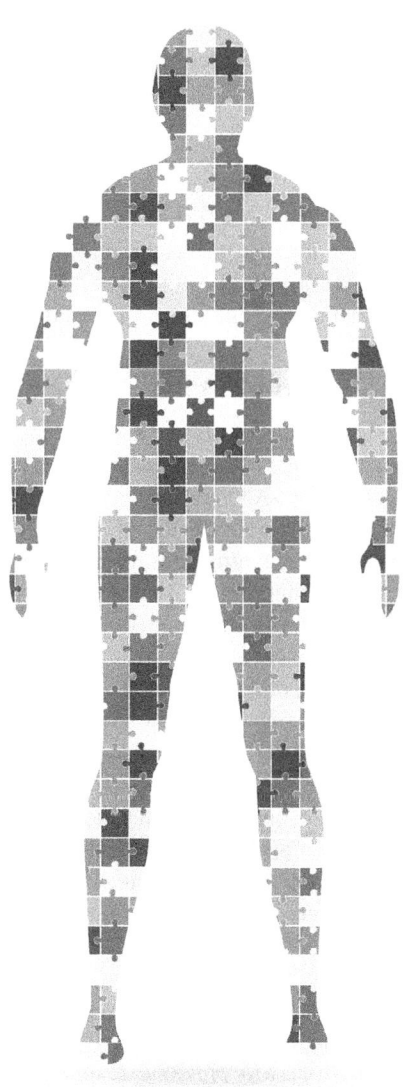

FIGURE 4.2 There are many more genes and biochemical pathways that interact to affect the functioning of MTHFR.

MTHFR (of which I gave an introductory definition in Chapter 1) is a small but mighty enzyme that the MTHFR gene produces that is involved in methylation, which is simply the transfer of a methyl group (CH3 [one carbon and three hydrogens]) from one place to another. There are dozens more enzymes directly involved in this pathway and hundreds indirectly involved.

Before I go into the functions of MTHFR, practitioners and real nerds like myself (What's up, my Nerdies?) may want to read over some basics of epigenetics in Appendix 4A. Some terms that are described are DNA structure, risk allele versus ancestral/"wild type" allele, upregulation (gain of function) and downregulation (loss of function), and why, as practitioners, we *cannot* and *must not* "treat the SNP." This can get drier and more boring than poorly cooked chicken breast, but I want to include it for context and because many practitioners want to or are starting to incorporate genetics into their practices.

I left some "good for the average reader to know" introductory information on genetics in the main text, but if you aren't interested in this, skim through and only digest the juicy nuggets that catch your attention until the action steps!

4.2 SINGLE NUCLEOTIDE POLYMORPHISMS

When a cell divides to make a new cell, its set of genetic instructions are copied. However, sometimes these instructions are copied incorrectly, like a typo, which leads to variations in the DNA sequence. Another analogy for a single nucleotide polymorphism is like incorrectly copying a recipe for an ingredient as "1 tsp" instead of "1 tbsp." Consequently, every time that erroneous recipe is copied, it will be "1 tsp." This is called a single nucleotide polymorphism. There is also data to support a premise that these genetic variations occur to confer some sort of survival or metabolic advantage, most probably due to adjustments to accommodate the dynamics of epigenetic factors. I will be referring to single nucleotide polymorphisms as SNPs throughout the book.

Single nucleotide polymorphisms are common variations that occur in human DNA. They are defined as having a greater than 1% incidence within the general population, although common polymorphisms can occur in up to 40–50% of the population.

SNPs occur, on average, in about one of every thousand nucleotides, which means there are roughly 4 to 5 million SNPs in any person's genome. Scientists have found more than 100 million SNPs in populations around the world. SNPs can also be used to track the inheritance of disease genes within families.

Most SNPs have no effect on health or development, but some have proven to impact our health greatly.

Again, knowing SNPs is not diagnostic, but it is indicative. I use them as a framework that allows me to craft a personalized protocol. Genetics can provide predictive information that helps determine why previous treatments may have been unsuccessful and what a better targeted treatment may be.

SNPs can affect our biochemical processes in almost endless ways. MedlinePlus. gov, part of the National Library of Medicine puts it succinctly:

> Researchers have found SNPs that may help predict an individual's response to certain drugs, susceptibility to environmental factors such as toxins, and risk of developing particular diseases.

4.3 ENZYMES REQUIRE NUTRITIONAL COFACTORS IN ORDER TO WORK

Cofactors are "helper" molecules that enzymes require in order to function. Genes make the blueprint for producing an enzyme. The gene gets transcribed into an enzyme, and the enzyme helps create a biochemical reaction. But the enzyme can only work if its required nutrients (vitamins, minerals, amino acids) are available, similar to specific types of fuel being needed to power different devices and machinery. I'd like to emphatically state again that *enzymes require nutritional cofactors in order to work*! This point is so nice, I've gotta say it twice.

One other point that I want to emphasize is that our bodies do not make minerals. If we don't consume them, our bodies won't have them to use! An inadequate intake of minerals forces the body to "rob Peter to pay Paul" by stealing minerals from other tissues in a sort of "hierarchy of needs." You can see how mineral deficiencies impair or prevent the body from being able to support a healthy pregnancy.

If we are talking about genes and genetic expression, we *have* to talk about nutrition. To not do so would be like talking about a sick fish and not discussing the water that it lives in or the food that it has been eating.

The enzymatic process can be inhibited by toxins, nutrient antagonists/deficiencies, stresses of all kinds, heavy metals, drugs, etc.

Various forms of stress inhibit enzymatic processes. This can be physical stress, mental and/or emotional stress, or oxidative stress (Figure 4.3).

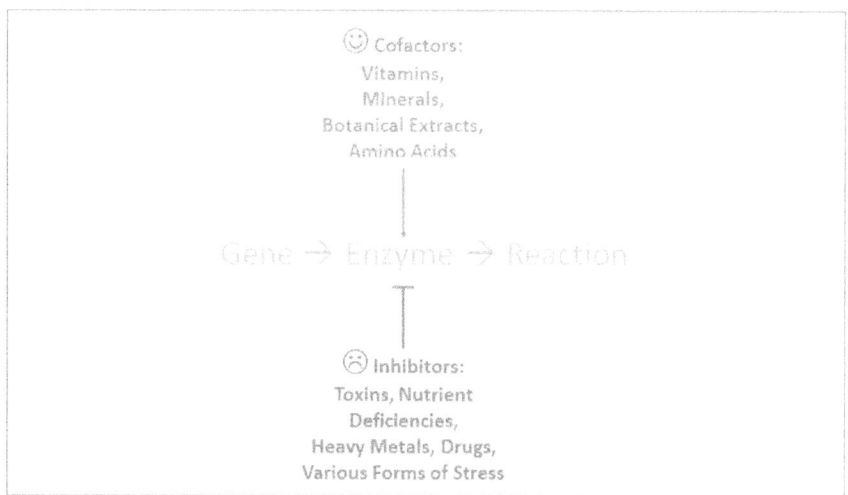

FIGURE 4.3 Enzymes require nutritional cofactors in order to work. Deficiencies, toxins, and stressors can inhibit enzyme activity.

Source: The author

4.4 EPIGENETICS DESCRIBES THE WAY THE GENOME INTERACTS WITH THE ENVIRONMENT

Epigenome, which literally means "on top of the genome," refers to all the factors that control how a gene is expressed. We are born with a set of DNA that, as far as is currently known, doesn't ever change. But our genetic expressions are like light switches, vulnerable to things that can switch them off and on. Actually, I like to think of genetic expression more like a dimmer switch, rather than a light switch, as there are fluctuating levels at which genes can be expressed.

Many people, even functional medicine professionals, often use the term "mutation" when referring to MTHFR or other genetic variants. Technically, a genetic mutation occurs in less than 1% of a population, whereas a single nucleotide polymorphism variant is seen to occur in more than 1% of a population. SNPs are the most common type of genetic variation among people.

Different from mutations, epigenetic changes lie not in the DNA itself, but in whether or not the genetic variants express and what actually causes them to express. You can boil it down to this differentiation: Genetics determines which genes you receive while epigenetics determines how those genes express. Mutations are essentially pathological changes in the gene that occur when the contextual environment in which the gene exists is deranged.

4.5 "GENETICS LOADS THE GUN, BUT ENVIRONMENT PULLS THE TRIGGER"

This is a popular phrase that describes epigenetics. SNPs can be caused by things like genetic adaptation (people living in Arctic regions or high elevations, for example), replication errors, errors in DNA repair, nutrient deficiencies, toxins, and radiation.

However, just because someone has a SNP does not mean it is doomed to express.

People think that there is nothing they can do about their disease risk, but we are not just what our genes are. We are our genes under the influence of our epigenome.

The presence of a particular gene or mutation in most cases merely connotes a predisposition to a particular biochemical activity, behavior, or disease process (Mead 2007: A582–A589). It has been estimated by the CDC that environmental and behavioral factors constitute roughly 90% of what determines whether a SNP will express. An article published in the Public Library of Science One (PLoS One) entitled "Genetic Factors Are Not the Major Causes of Chronic Diseases" details these claims, noting that chronic disease is only 16.4% genetic and 84.6% environmental. (Rappaport 2016) This means that our mindset and emotions, our diet, our stress levels, our nutrient status, and our exposure to toxins in food, water, and air all play a much bigger part in our disease risk (and fertility) than does our genetics. In fact, environmental and social stressors are the primary source of epigenetic modifications. (Rozanov 2012) And most of that starts with the food we choose to eat every day.

4.6 FOOD AND ENVIRONMENT ARE INFORMATION FOR OUR GENES

Numerous studies in humans, animals, and cell cultures have demonstrated a wide array of food constituents that can influence and/or regulate gene expression in diverse ways, including hormonal balance, immune system robustness, and detoxification processes. The same goes for toxin exposures, altering the functionality of genes and how they express.

A perfect example of epigenetics is identical twins. They are born with the exact same DNA. As they get older, they make more of their own life choices and they become less and less "identical." Differing diets, stressors, and toxin exposures will act as genetic operators, flipping on and off the expression of the genes. One twin will weigh more or have more wrinkles than the other, or one twin will get diabetes while the other gets cancer (Figure 4.4).

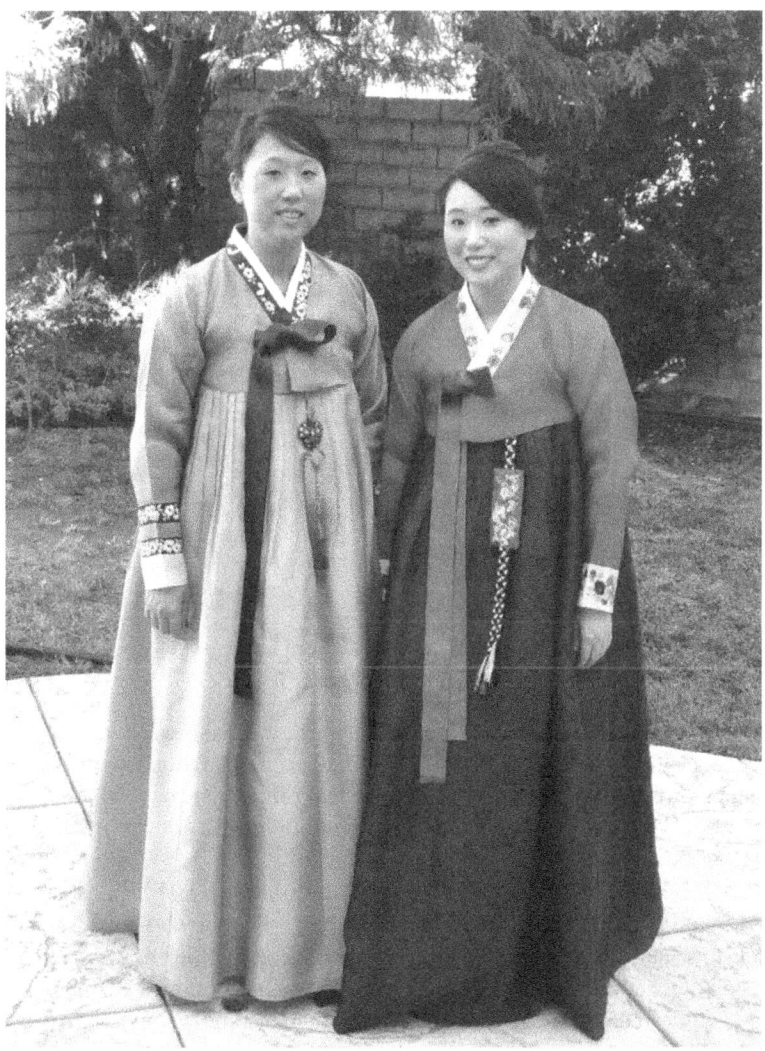

FIGURE 4.4   Photo of long-lost identical twins who were separated at birth in Korea and each adopted by a different family in the United States. Reunited after 33 years.

Source: Katey Bennett and Amanda Dunford

4.7 GOVERNMENT NUTRITION RECOMMENDATIONS ARE ANTIQUATED

The Recommended Dietary Allowance (RDA) levels were replaced with the Recommended Dietary Reference Intake levels (RDI) following the passage of the Dietary Supplement and Health Education Act (DSHEA) of 1994. These levels are set by the Institute of Medicine and are considered to be the daily amount of nutrients needed to prevent the development of diseases and death due to nutrient deficiencies. Differing needs may have been taken into consideration between gender, age, and whether a woman is pregnant or breastfeeding. Outside these parameters, nutrition science has traditionally focused on the assumption that all individuals have the same basic nutritional requirements, just like the pharmaceutical industry model of "one drug fits all." Thankfully, however, this paradigm is changing.

The RDI levels are definitely not the levels of nutrients needed for optimal nourishment and functioning. They are merely the amount needed to prevent diseases of deficiency. The RDI is updated periodically to reflect new knowledge, but it is undeniable that chronic diseases related to nutrition have been increasing in recent years (Fenech et al. 2011).

The RDI has not been optimized for genetic subgroups that may greatly vary in the activity of transport, absorption, utilization, or metabolism of a micronutrient and/or the enzymes that require that micronutrient as a cofactor. That's where the field of nutrigenomics is so helpful! We can easily see where someone may have a greater need for a nutrient due to variations in genes related to transport or utilization of that particular nutrient.

Nutrigenomics is blazing the trail for personalized functional nutrition. It is essentially the study of the effects of nutrients on our individual genetic expression and how that can protect the genome from damage and maintain genomic integrity.

4.8 NOW THAT YOU KNOW ALL THAT, IT'S FINALLY TIME TO TALK ABOUT MTHFR

Remember that I stated that genes are the blueprint for making enzymes. MTHFR is a gene that provides coding for the production of an enzyme called methylenetetrahydrofolate reductase (MTHFR). It plays a critical role in the conversion of synthetic folic acid into methylfolate, the form that the body is able to use (the bioavailable form). It also has many other functions.

The MTHFR variant is probably the most well-known, and it plays a huge part in how folate is used and metabolized in the body. People who have MTHFR polymorphisms have some degree of decreased conversion efficiency. As I stated earlier, receiving a copy from one parent (heterozygous) can reduce enzyme efficiency 20–40% while receiving copies from both parents (homozygous) can reduce efficiency up to 70%.

Folic acid is not naturally found in food! It is a synthetic nutrient that has been made in a laboratory. Folate is the form that is found in foliage like leafy greens, as well as eggs, liver, and other fruits and vegetables. Folic acid (as opposed to the bioavailable folate form) is found in some supplements and in refined grains and other fortified foods like cereal and breads.

A note on fortification: Processed and refined foods are stripped of their nutrients during processing, and the government requires that they be put back in. Only a fraction of what has been taken out is put back in, and many of those forms are synthetic and not ideal forms for the body to be able to utilize. This punctuates the importance of eating a naturally wholesome, nutrient-rich and nourishing diet.

Synthetic folic acid is lacking the body's most fundamental biochemical compound – a methyl group (simply, a carbon with three hydrogens attached – CH_3). Methyl groups are passed back and forth to make all sorts of things happen in the body, in every cell and every organ, every instant of the day. It is said that methylation (the transfer of a methyl group) takes place o*ver 1 billion times per second!* Many highly regarded doctors and practitioners have stated this in their blogs. However, when I tried to find the source for that statement, I didn't have a whole lot of luck. Either way, methylation is critical for us to live.

Since roughly half of the world's population has an MTHFR variant (prevalence varies among ethnicities), potentially compromising folic acid utilization, supplementing with and fortifying foods with folic acid doesn't seem like a beneficial choice.

4.9 FOLIC ACID CONVERSION TO FOLATE

To convert folic acid into methylfolate requires multiple functional genes producing functional enzymes, which require adequate cofactors.

But that is only half of it. Enzyme production and activity can also be inhibited by toxins. Enzymes must be produced in an environment free of compounds that interfere with their function, such as heavy metals, toxic chemicals, and some medications.

There are other genes in the methylation pathway that can be variated and, when combined with an MTHFR variant, can make the conversion efficiency of folic acid into methylfolate even worse. Deficiencies in nutritional cofactors can further compound this conversion, adding insult to injury. Some genetic variants in the methylation pathway have been associated with neural tube defects (Parle-McDermott et al. 2006) and pregnancy loss. Refer to Appendix 4B to see a diagram of the steps and genes involved in turning folic acid into methylfolate. Unless you are a practitioner, you likely have no reason to learn the associated genes or be interested in the diagram. I just wanted to include them to emphasize the point that MTHFR is but a small part of a larger pathway.

As previously mentioned, deficiencies in cofactors can impair methylation. For example, a deficiency in choline in a pregnant mother can cause genetic changes in the offspring. Choline is the crucial building material needed for fetal brain and nervous system development. A sufficient supply of dietary choline is necessary for optimum development of the fetus and breast-fed infants (Smallwood et al. 2016). For more detailed information about the importance of choline and the commonly variated PEMT gene that produces it, please refer to Chapter 10, "The Importance of Proper Fat Utilization for Hormonal Balance and Fetal Growth."

Low conversion ability from any of the polymorphisms combined with a high intake of synthetic folic acid can lead to a high level of unmetabolized folic acid in the body (Smith et al. 2008), which has been linked to health problems (Powers 2007) like decreases in natural killer cell activity (Troen et al. 2006) and cancer. It can also mask a B12 deficiency.

Unmetabolized folic acid has no physiological benefit to the host until it is converted into dihydrofolate by the DHFR gene. So, if you have MTHFR and/or DHFR variants, or if you don't know what your MTHFR status is, it's probably wise to steer clear of folic acid. It is best not to be eating those refined and fortified grains if whole foods are available anyway.

4.10 METHYLFOLATE

Methylfolate is the methylated form of folate, which is also called vitamin B9.

It is involved in many essential bodily functions, such as:

- Making and repairing DNA
- Helping convert homocysteine (a marker of health and reproductive risk) back into the amino acid methionine
- Neurotransmitter production
- Producing platelets and red and white blood cells
- Growing a fetus
- DNA expression/silencing (turning genes on and off)
- Proper immune system functioning (building T and NK cells)
- Supporting myelination of neurons
- Detoxification (especially of heavy metals)
- Energy production
- Metabolizing hormones
- Production of antioxidants

Methylfolate drives the body's ever-important methylation pathway.

The simple definition of methylation as it pertains to DNA is the addition of a methyl group (CH_3) to DNA. Methylation (or lack thereof) affects genetic expression and integrity and enables a gene to turn on or off by the transfer of a methyl group.

Methylation affects numerous other pathways and cycles in the body, including the urea cycle and the Krebs cycle, which is responsible for energy production. Methylation is also a phase 2 liver detoxification pathway, so it is important for clearing hormones and toxins from the body.

Rather than reducing MTHFR (or any SNP for that matter) to a single problem that needs one nutrient to help compensate, it is crucial to look at groups of SNPs or, even more importantly, entire biochemical pathways and the diet/lifestyle of the person to determine a route of action. The SNPs just give clues as to what could be causing an issue.

It is important to point out that a person can have problems with methylation without any related genetic mutations.

B vitamins are essential cofactors for the methylation pathway. Remember that I said that enzymes can't work without cofactors. If we are deficient in B12 or folate, the methylation cycle won't spin efficiently.

Certain drugs can inhibit gene activity and/or rob the body of methylation ability, whether they deplete B12, folate, or any other cofactor needed in the pathway. Some of these drugs are estrogen, methotrexate, metformin, and nitrous oxide. In these cases, methylation function is impaired because of a drug, not because of your genes.

The same goes with toxins. Certain toxins and heavy metals interfere with methylation ability. Most people think of toxins as harmful synthetic chemical compounds that are found in the modern day. While those are a very serious and excessive occurrence, we cannot forget the mold and mycotoxins that are biotoxins which have been around since the beginning of time. In Chapter 7, I discuss how mold and mycotoxins inhibit fertility and why they are much more of a problem now than in the past.

If I could count how many times I've heard people say that they are on methylfolate (and oftentimes incredibly large doses) because they have MTHFR, I wouldn't have gotten this book written because I'd still be trying to add them up.

When I work with clients and train practitioners, I emphasize that MTHFR is often the *last* block that should be placed on the metaphorical and literal (Functional Genomic Analysis) support pyramid (which I describe in Appendix 1A), after all foundations have been laid securely in place. Refer to Appendix 4C for the reasons and why we should not start supplementing with methylfolate without making sure other important foundations are in place.

My colleagues and I have seen an all-too-common scenario way too many times. Clients will come to us after their previous practitioner had them start supplementing with folate, on which they felt great for two weeks as their deficiency was being addressed, but then they crashed hard and experienced crazy agitation or anxiety once it got the metabolic cogs spinning. Folate is definitely needed but not until other foundational needs are addressed first (like issues with the glutathione pathway, antioxidant production, iron dysregulation, etc.), which I will be discussing. *Again, this is why someone cannot solely test for MTHFR and treat the SNP.*

I always use the analogy with my clients that we must first put out the fire before we clean the house and start rebuilding. Folate is a rebuilding, repairing nutrient, which is why it is critical for a healthy pregnancy.

So you see, when you don't address inflammatory factors and detoxification first, supporting MTHFR can backfire.

This is why we do not treat the SNPs.

4.11 NOTES ON INTERMITTENT FASTING

Intermittent fasting has risen in popularity in the past few years. If you're not familiar, it involves eating only within a certain window of time each day. For some, that's a 12-hour window, and for seasoned fasters, it's 4 hours or even less.

The reason intermittent fasting offers many great benefits to the body is because it allows the body to flip into a state of autophagy (refer to Appendix 4C for information on autophagy and mTOR, including a visual) while not allowing it to feel the stress of a complete fast. Autophagy occurs when cells can go into repair mode because they don't have growth factors coming in, like proteins or sugars, for example. The cells start to "digest" their own undesirable contents, which cleans up the cells, allowing them to work more efficiently. If there are constant, incoming growth factors, the cell is stuck in growth mode. If the growth factors are excessive and the cell does not have time to "clean house," then aberrant growth happens, causing things like tumors, cysts, stones, and endometriosis. If autophagy doesn't take place, inflammation will set in and create a whole host of undesirable possibilities, and as I stated in the first paragraphs of this book, inflammation is a primary component of impaired fertility.

Many people don't understand that there are many things that promote cellular growth besides food, like pesticides and plastics. I also know plenty of people who are practicing intermittent fasting but are still taking growth-promoting supplements like methylfolate, iron, and glutamine, which interrupt or block the autophagy process.

It is important to allow your body to go through anabolic (growth) and catabolic (breaking down/cleaning) cycles. I think this is exemplified through our human history of feast and famine.

This is where pulsing supplements can work in your favor.

An example of a week of pulsing for autophagy promotion would look like three or four days of intermittent fasting with moderate aerobic exercise, meals free of animal products (amino acids, as well as hormones from conventional, factory farmed/concentrated [or confined] animal feeding operations [CAFO] meat and dairy, promote mTOR) and your mTOR-blocking, autophagy-promoting supplements. The other three or four days would be your strength training exercises, bone broth, and animal-based foods, coupled with your rebuilding/repairing supplements like folate and l-glutamine. I say three or four days because we all have different growth/cleanup needs depending on age, activity levels, health history, etc.

As you'll read in the upcoming pages, detox ability is far more than just MTHFR and methylation.

Methylation is a phase 2 liver detox pathway. In addition to methylation, some other phase 2 liver detox pathways are acetylation, glucuronidation, and glutathione conjugation, which are made possible by the genes that produce the enzymes to drive those reactions, *if* they have the necessary cofactors and are not inhibited by toxins. I will be discussing these other detox pathways in the pages and chapters ahead.

When the body's cells, tissues, organs, and systems are healthy, cells effectively and efficiently make energy, manage that energy, and eliminate cellular wastes (we'll call them "cellular dirty diapers") constantly. Once again, while inflammation can be a normal protective response, the inflammation itself is not the problem; it is what's *causing* the inflammation that is the underlying problem. Most people alive today are bombarded with all sorts of stuff that impairs cellular functioning and promotes inflammation. Inflammation is a sign that detoxification could be impaired to some extent and needs to be fixed. In my observation, the detoxification ability of our cells, organs, and systems may actually be more important than diet these days. I talk all about toxins and ways to detoxify them in Chapter 12 and Chapter 13, respectively. However, nourishing the cellular ability to make energy, managing that energy, and then being able to eliminate toxins by opening up drainage pathways (collectively called "cell metabolism"), should be the strategic priority before trying to purge toxic/waste materials from cells and organs. Doing a detox program *after* addressing this most important first step will reduce the potential of a harsh detox/cleansing reaction, called a Herxheimer reaction. Keep in mind, the mechanism of action for many purgative products (purging agents like butcher's broom, yellow dock, blessed thistle, wild Oregon grape, dandelion root, psyllium seed husks, senna, etc.) is to irritate the tissue to "force" the purging of toxins from those already toxic/fragile metabolically impaired tissues/organs: e.g., the GI tract, liver, kidneys, spleen, gallbladder, etc. This means that toxins are being released and exposed to other weakened tissues. If the systems/tissues are weak, the toxins purged from those tissues will almost certainly not be able to be completely eliminated, meaning that the toxins will circulate and be reabsorbed into fragile tissues. This is what generally causes the most significant and harshest Herxheimer reactions. In fact, in many cases, greater fatigue will be the primary detox symptom because the immune system works hardest while you sleep and will be compelling you to get some sleep so it can cleanse, repair, regenerate, and rejuvenate your cell, tissue, organ, and systems functions. That's why, when you are healthier, you have a bowel movement after awakening in the morning: getting rid of the toxic wastes.

4.12 ACTION STEPS FOR PATIENTS

- Be sure to nourish the body to ensure proper genetic cofactor availability. Refer to the next chapter, "Eat a *Nourishing* Diet, Not a 'Healthy' Diet," to learn what this entails.
- Do a salivary genetic test kit. As I previously stated, 23andMe was what my colleagues and I used prior to the chip change in 2017, when they took out thousands of SNPs that we found relevant for analysis. Since this chip change, many businesses and practitioners have created their own chips. I personally use and recommend the Your Functional Genomics (YFG)[2] salivary test kit because it includes more genetic SNPs in metabolic pathways than just the clinically researched ones that many genetic testing companies include. Just because an SNP hasn't been researched yet doesn't mean it isn't significant. This kit will already have the SNPs included if/when the research comes out.
- Upload your raw genetic data to a genetic interpretation software. Every single one has a different array of genes, with some "standard" genes being included in all of them. Some of the genes I mention in this book may not be in other software or part of a salivary test kit. While there are some really great interpretation services and software out there (the results of which many clients share with me), I personally use Functional Genomic Analysis.[3]

NOTES

1 Functional genomics, as defined in the *Encyclopedia of Bioinformatics and Computational Biology* (2019), is a branch that integrates molecular biology and cell biology studies and deals with the whole structure, function and, regulation of a gene (and the proteins they produce) in contrast to the gene-by-gene approach of classical molecular biology technique.

2 I do not receive any financial compensation for this recommendation. This is just my personal preference and the one I am most familiar with.

3 As I stated in the introduction, I am available for interpretation services and consultations for both practitioners and clients for genomic interpretation.

REFERENCES

Fenech, Michael, Ahmed El-Sohemy, Leah Cahill, Lynnette R. Ferguson, Tapaeru-Ariki C. French, E. Shyong Tai, John Milner, et al. 2011. "Nutrigenetics and nutrigenomics: viewpoints on the current status and applications in nutrition research and practice." *Lifestyle Genomics* 4, no. 2, 68–69.

Mead, M. Nathaniel. 2007. "Nutrigenomics: the genome – food interface." *Environmental Health Perspectives* 115, no. 12, A582–A589.

Parle-McDermott, Anne, Peadar N. Kirke, James L. Mills, Anne M. Molloy, Christopher Cox, Valerie B. O'Leary, Faith Pangilinan, et al. 2006. "Confirmation of the R653Q polymorphism of the trifunctional C1-synthase enzyme as a maternal risk for neural tube defects in the Irish population." *European Journal of Human Genetics* 14, no. 6, 768–772.

Powers, Hilary J. 2007. "Folic acid under scrutiny." *British Journal of Nutrition* 98, no. 4, 665–666.

Rappaport, Stephen M. 2016. "Genetic factors are not the major causes of chronic diseases." *PLoS One* 11, no. 4, e0154387.

Rozanov, V. A. 2012. "Epigenetics: stress and behavior." *Neurophysiology* 44, no. 4, 332–350.

Smallwood, Tangi, Hooman Allayee, and Brian J. Bennett. 2016. "Choline metabolites: gene by diet interactions." *Current Opinion in Lipidology* 27, no. 1, 33.

Smith, A. David, Young-In Kim, and Helga Refsum. 2008. "Is folic acid good for everyone?" *The American Journal of Clinical Nutrition* 87, no. 3, 517–533.

Troen, Aron M., Breeana Mitchell, Bess Sorensen, Mark H. Wener, Abbey Johnston, Brent Wood, Jacob Selhub, et al. 2006. "Unmetabolized folic acid in plasma is associated with reduced natural killer cell cytotoxicity among postmenopausal women." *The Journal of Nutrition* 136, no. 1, 189–194.

5 Eat a *Nourishing* Diet, Not a "Healthy" Diet

This is where it all begins! This is what our bodies have evolved to function and thrive on. Keep in mind that you are made of only air, water, food, and sunshine. The quality of those resources and the ability of the body to use them determine the quality of your health and metabolism.

When discussing food, I tell my clients, "There are only two types of food: Food that nourishes the body, and food that burdens it." What this looks like for each individual varies widely, but all bodies need nourishment. I highly recommend working with a functional nutrition practitioner to determine what that means for *your* body.[1] However, the tips and action steps in this chapter will provide you with some solid information to get you on the right track. We don't want to just eat "healthy" foods; we want a variety of nourishing foods that offer a diverse array of nutrients as well as food for our microbiome/gut health. "Healthy" is a word that has been bastardized and is thrown around almost as much as the term "all natural" in the food industry. There is little to no regulation of the use of these words on food packages or in advertising, and they definitely may not be nourishing to the body.

It is interesting to note that nutrient deficiencies are common. A 2017 study found that over 30% of Americans have at least one vitamin deficiency (Bird et al. 2017), with deficiency risk being higher in women, and that percentage increases as socioeconomic status decreases. One reason for nutrient deficiencies being so prevalent nowadays may be the fact that the food grown today is significantly lower in nutrient content than the food our grandparents ate (Davis et al. 2004).

However, nourishment does not reside only in the realm of food. Emotional and spiritual (not limited to religion) nourishment are just as important. I discuss these aspects in the next chapter.

The main thing to know regarding a healthy diet is to *just eat real food*. Not food with flavor enhancers, texturizers, stabilizers, dyes, preservatives, added sugars, pesticides, fungicides, herbicides, antibiotics, hormones, or food that has been processed. These substances are used to make food taste better, look better, be bigger, and last longer for commercial viability; it's all about the money! Remember in Chapter 4, I described how genes make enzymes, and those enzymes require nutritional cofactors in order to work? Whole, nourishing foods are where those nutritional cofactors ideally come from. Our livers were not designed to have to deal with all that garbage in our food, on top of all the other chemicals and toxins out there in our environment. This is where preparing meals to nourish your body is necessary. Remember in Chapter 1, I shared how self-care involves putting in the hard work? This is the epitome of self-care and care for your future children. Make it a priority to take the time to prepare clean, nourishing meals.

DOI: 10.1201/b23201-7

Convenience is killing us and our earth. Prioritizing the time and money it takes to buy and prepare nourishing food will result in much better health, happiness, and fertility than, say, always binge-watching the latest Netflix show. I often hear people say, "Buying organic food is expensive." No, missing work or experiencing substandard work output because you feel like crap is expensive. Designer handbags are expensive and don't serve you in the way that nourishing food does. I personally find health to be much sexier than designer clothes and bags anyway. Cancer and diabetes are expensive and life degrading, so pay the farmer now, or pay the pharmacy later. Buy as much organic food as is affordable, at least the foods you eat most often.

I want to note that, for many years in my past, my income qualified me for government assistance. I am fully aware of the socioeconomic divide that can make buying "health foods" cost prohibitive. Frozen vegetables are often much cheaper than fresh vegetables. And frozen vegetables are cheaper than buying packaged foods. There are ways that people in food deserts have made it possible to eat a healthful diet with community gardens, seed sharing, container planting, buying in bulk (dried legumes, grains, etc.), and cooking from scratch. Check out the Food is Free Project and the awesome, inspiring things they are doing and sharing in communities across the world.

- Action step: Buy local! Food that is grown in your local area will often contain a higher nutrient profile than food that has been transported long distances. This is due to the fact that food that is transported long distances must be picked before it is ripe, whereas local produce is able to ripen in the soil or on the tree/vine, allowing the full nutrient profile to develop. Also, as harvested food sits, it can decrease in nutrients and phytochemicals. Consider joining a local community-supported agriculture (CSA) group or shopping at your local farmer's market.

5.1 WATER NOURISHES THE BODY AND IS ESSENTIAL FOR LIFE

Up to 60% of the human adult body is water. In fact, according to USGS.gov, the brain and heart are composed of 73% water, and the lungs are about 83% water. The skin contains 64% water, muscles and kidneys are 79%, and even the bones are watery: 31%. (USGS 2019) Let's hope that the water we drink is clean and clear of toxins.

In a Before the Bump (i.e., pre-pregnancy) workshop I created years ago, I asked attendees to think about all the cleaners that are under their kitchen/bathroom sinks and under the sinks of everyone on their street, in their neighborhood, and in their town and state. And then think about how long those cleaners have been getting poured out or rinsed down the drain by all these homes for decades. All those cleaners end up in our water supply, along with pesticide and herbicide runoff from lawns and farms; car chemicals; factory waste; urinary excretion of birth control hormones, chemotherapy drugs, antidepressants, and antibiotics; etc. This alone is a call to action to be more vigilant about what you are exposed to and how these products can adversely affect your health.

- Action step: Tap water for drinking, cooking, and bathing *must* be filtered with a quality filter. If you use reverse osmosis (which is my preference), I highly recommend remineralizing it. Although the water is clean, it is lacking minerals, which can cause imbalances in the body. Minerals maintain correct pH in the body. The best countertop RO filtration system I've seen so far is the Aqua-Tru (see Resources section for more info). However, if a countertop reverse osmosis filter is not in your budget at the moment, I have two other recommendations. The first is a Zero Water filter. This filter comes with a cool testing stick that measures the total dissolved solids in water so you know when to change the filter. I recommend remineralizing Zero Water as well since it's so good at taking things out of the water that some of the minerals may also be filtered out. The second option is to refill large jugs at water-filling stations, which is usually RO water. I know most five-gallon jugs are plastic, but there's less surface area for the plastic to leach, especially if you get new jugs often. Also, these jugs are harder plastic than your smaller water bottles, so they aren't as quickly prone to leach. Remember, we're striving for progress through a "this is better than that" approach, not perfection. A third and final option, if you can make the investment, is to install an RO filtration system, which gets integrated right into your water supply to your house.

Another huge step to ensure your body is nourished is to avoid refined sugar. Refined sugar is an antinutrient, which is why I'm discussing it in this chapter, rather than in the toxins chapter. An "anti-nutrient" is a substance that blocks the absorption of nutrients and/or requires more resources to be metabolized and cleared than it provides; it's more of a burden than a benefit. Aside from being tasty, sugar has *zero* redeeming value. I don't consider its high calorie and carbohydrate content a win since there are nourishing ways to get those.

Sugar can affect proper gut functioning, pH maintenance, and hormone balance because it encourages the overgrowth of fungi, parasites, and bacteria, and it decreases the colonization of healthy bacteria.

Sugar contributes to insulin resistance, blood sugar abnormalities, and obesity, not just from caloric means but also because it is pro-inflammatory and sends the body into a mild "state of alarm," (a.k.a. "survival panic") and energy conservation and can cause hormonal disruption, which leads to obesity. Historically, fat was survival insurance, and our biological reactivity hasn't changed much in tens of thousands of years. Obesity and the inflammation associated with it have been linked to reproductive issues and complications.

Sugar is just tasty poison!

- Action step: My recommendation for you would be to try a sugar detox. While the goal is not necessarily to stop eating sugar forever, doing a sugar detox will help you balance your blood sugar, lose weight, cool off inflammation, improve digestion, and reset your palate to be more sensitive to sugar. After a sugar detox, things will taste a lot sweeter than before. In Chapter 15, I write about how blood sugar imbalances derail hormones and can lead to polycystic ovary syndrome (PCOS) and other fertility challenges. I also mention some supplements that can be taken to improve insulin/blood sugar management in that chapter.

To ensure adequate nourishment, supplements are often used to help "move the needle" faster than diet alone. Keep in mind that they are called "supplements" not "substitutes." You can't supplement your way out of a poor diet.

Knowing which supplements to purchase is overwhelming. The topic of supplements can get very individualized, but the bottom line here is that whatever supplements you choose, try to make sure they are made with integrity. This is often a very tough thing for the average consumer to decipher, so I wanted to provide you with the basics.

I judge the quality of a supplement based on the form of the nutrient that is used, just like I judge a restaurant based on the type of lettuce they use in their salads. If a restaurant only offers iceberg lettuce as a salad option, they either don't know what a quality salad is, or they use the cheapest ingredients just to have a salad on the menu. And they probably use anemic-looking tomatoes that lack flavor to accompany it!

The same goes with supplements. Deciding which vitamins to buy is confusing for lots of people, and making a wrong choice can cause you to, quite literally, waste your money. If your vitamins can't be used by the body, they're doing you about as much good as if you'd put them in your pocket instead of your mouth. Actually, for many of the supplements that you buy at big box chain stores, putting them in your pocket may actually be safer than swallowing them.

5.2 HERE ARE SOME BASIC TIPS TO KNOW IF A SUPPLEMENT IS HALFWAY DECENT

Look at the "other ingredients" list. If there's an extensive paragraph situation goin' on, ditch it. If there are food dyes, hydrogenated oils, polyethylene glycol, non-organic soy or corn,[2] it's going to tax your body more than it will help it.

The second easiest way to tell if your supplement is *el cheapo* is if the form of calcium used is calcium carbonate. This is chalk; it's limestone. Our bodies weren't designed to eat rocks, so why put them into a supplement? Because it's the cheapest form of calcium, that's why! With supplements, you usually get what you pay for.

Here's another tidbit about calcium. It needs the help of other nutrients, called cofactors, in order to be taken into the bones. Unless your diet or supplement contains vitamin K2 (which ushers calcium into the bones) and other nutrients like vitamin D3, magnesium, strontium, and/or vanadium, the calcium you supplement with may be getting deposited willy-nilly in soft tissue, like arterial walls. Rather than supplementing with calcium, eat more leafy greens with pastured butter (rich in vitamin K2) and canned wild salmon and sardines with the bones, which you can easily mash and are anti-inflammatory and great for brain health to boot. When you do this, you get all the forms and cofactors you need.

- Action steps:
  ○ Avoid buying supplements at the big box chain stores.
  ○ Look for supplements that use minimal "other ingredients."

○ Try to avoid minerals that are "rock salts" (like calcium carbonate and/ or calcium phosphate, just to name a couple). That means that a mineral is bound to another mineral and is essentially a ground-up rock. (When was the last time you ate some good old rocks?)

○ Look for patents and trademarks in the supplement facts or ingredient list. These often represent science-based premium quality ingredients used in the formula. Look for real science and scientific validation with references, like I have used in this book.

NOTES

1 If you don't have one, find one! You can also connect with me through social media (IG: @ FunctionalFertilitySolutions) or my website, JaclynDowns.com, for valuable information and other resources/references.

2 Soy and corn are the most highly genetically modified crops aside from cotton. If they aren't labeled organic, they are very likely genetically modified and sprayed with pesticides and herbicides with reckless abandon. For more about the health effects of GMOs on our future generations, refer to the blog I wrote on my website, JaclynDowns.com.

REFERENCES

Bird, Julia K., Rachel A. Murphy, Eric D. Ciappio, and Michael I. McBurney. 2017. "Risk of deficiency in multiple concurrent micronutrients in children and adults in the United States." *Nutrients* 9, no. 7, 655.

Davis, Donald R., Melvin D. Epp, and Hugh D. Riordan. 2004. "Changes in USDA food composition data for 43 garden crops, 1950 to 1999." *Journal of the American College of Nutrition* 23, no. 6, 669–682.

USGS. 2019. *USGS.gov*, May 22. www.usgs.gov/special-topic/water-science-school/science/ water-you-water-and-human-body?qt-science_center_objects=0#qt-science_center_objects.

6 Address Stress: Your Physical and Emotional Health May Be Hindering Your Fertility

There are so many genetic and biochemical variations between us that everyone's needs are different. However, there certainly are things that are beneficial for *all* humans, and I'll even venture to say all creatures, regardless of genetics. These are foundations for health that pertain to everyone. If these foundations are not implemented, all the supplements and protocols in the world will only take you so far, but you will not cross the threshold into optimal wellness, vitality, and fertility.

Within this chapter are my foundational guidelines for optimal wellness, complete with actionable suggestions you can implement right away. These are things I address with each client. They are foundational steps that can, when implemented, expedite your desired wellness and/or fertility outcomes, and can even negate the need to engage in significantly deeper protocols. These lifestyle suggestions will allow a full functional approach for proper epigenetic expression, even without knowing your genetic profile.

The limbic system has a direct effect on the nervous and endocrine systems. In Chapter 1, I introduced and defined the limbic system and psychoneuroimmunology. As part of the limbic system, the hypothalamic-pituitary-adrenal (HPA) axis will inhibit reproductive function when activated by stressors.

The HPA axis is a signaling pathway between your brain and the system of glands and hormones that are central to the metabolic system, immune functions, behavior, stress response, and reproduction. The HPA axis directly affects the function of the thyroid gland, as well as the adrenal glands and gonads. As a quick recap of what I wrote in Chapter 1, when the hypothalamus perceives stress, it signals the pituitary gland to tell the adrenal glands to release cortisol and adrenaline (epinephrine). This is what happens when we move into the sympathetic nervous system response of "fight or flight." Historically, the stressor was a predator; our "fight or flight" response kicked in to get us out of a dangerous situation. Once we moved to safety or the situation was resolved, the stress hormones stopped being produced and we switched back into our parasympathetic "rest, digest, repair, reproduce" mode, also referred to as the "feed and breed" state.

Remember that any kind of stress can cause the limbic system and HPA axis to get dysregulated. Those stressors are what this whole book is about. So in this chapter, I want to give you some tools that help keep the body in a parasympathetic state to optimize reproductive capabilities.

DOI: 10.1201/b23201-8

ACTION STEPS

- Get outdoors. Our bodies thrive on fresh air, preferably within nature. Oxygen is vital for our bodies to function. We are made of nothing else but air, water, food, and sunshine. The quality of our health is determined by the quality of those resources and our cellular ability to use them effectively and efficiently to create and maintain the ideal biological environment. Our intimate relationship with the earth and its water, air, and sunshine is crucial. The importance of a "thing" can be determined by how long you live without it. Air wins! I discuss the importance of this more in the section ahead on mindful breathing.
- Nature and grounding. So much of our human existence has been outside in nature. Our feet were directly on and in the earth; we slept on the earth; we were constantly exposed to good microbes in the earth. We evolved being grounded on the earth. It makes sense that being close to nature is what grounds us, and it does, literally and figuratively. I like the way the late Dr. Stephen Sinatra, a world-renowned cardiologist, explained the science of grounding: "Just like the earth, your body is mostly water and minerals, and both are excellent conductors of electrons. We are bioelectrical beings living on an electrical planet." This may sound like something that only crunchy hippies will endorse, but there are, indeed, articles in scientific journals on the benefits of grounding (earthing). Biophysicists, electrical engineers, and experts in electrophysiology and geophysics can explain the science of it. The bottom line is that grounding reduces stress, anxiety, depression, pain, and inflammation and resynchronizes cortisol secretion more in alignment with the naturally 24-hour circadian rhythm profile. Remember that I stated earlier in the book that cortisol dysregulation is a contributing factor to impaired fertility? The authors of one study explain that the earth's ground is rife with negatively charged electrons that act as antioxidants in the body, with zero negative secondary effects, because our body evolved to use them over eons of physical contact with the ground. They state, "Our immune systems work beautifully as long as electrons are available to balance the ROS and reactive nitrogen species (RNS) [types of free radicals that cause inflammation] used when dealing with infection and tissue injury. Our modern lifestyle has taken the body and the immune system by surprise by suddenly depriving it of its primordial electron source" (Oschman et al. 2015).
  - Fun fact: You can see evidence of the earth's negative charge! We all know that negative charges repel each other, which you can witness when playing with magnets. Oxygen carries a negative charge, and therefore, the surface of a water molecule does as well (H_2'O'). This negatively charged repelling is what causes heavy rain clouds, rife with water, to stay up in the air. This is also why they appear to be flat on the bottom. The earth and rain clouds repel each other, rather than the clouds just magically 'floating' in the sky. So, to sum it up,

get grounded to reduce pain and inflammation, improve mood and sleep, and stabilize your physiology, all of which are beneficial for fertility.

- Sunshine. We are designed to thrive on sunshine. We are solar-powered beings; sunlight may even help the skin produce serotonin (Sansone and Sansone 2013). The skin, the largest organ of the body, is not the only part of the body that reacts to the sun's rays. The retinas in our eyes are photo-sensitive and connect directly to various parts of the brain, activating many biochemical and biophysical reactions in the body. These reactions include stimulating the hypothalamus and pituitary glands, which are the head hon-chos in charge of adrenal functioning, hormone production and secretion, and stimulating the pineal gland that requires darkness at night and enough full spectrum daylight to regulate circadian rhythm. We evolved to wake with the sun and be outside much of the time. Our bodies knew what time it was long before clocks and watches, and our bodies depend on this innate sensing for optimal health.

- Manage stress. Since it will always be easier to say "get rid of stress" than to actually make that happen, I prefer utilizing stress management tools. Since the central principle of this book is how stressors from various sources dis-rupt the autonomic nervous system (and the limbic system that regulates it) and hinder reproductive capacity, I certainly wanted to include a few action-able ways to support autonomic nervous system (ANS) balance.

  - Guided relaxation is a nice alternative for people who find meditation difficult to do. This is usually done with someone guiding you to tune in to each of the different parts of your body, generally starting from the head down to the toes, implementing conscious relaxation. There are a ton of recordings of various lengths out there (lots on YouTube), so experiment with a few and find some you like.

  - Self-care. My definition of self-care isn't "pampering yourself" with pedicures and chocolate. Self-care is creating wellness for yourself physically, mentally, and emotionally. It is putting in the work to ensure you create a life that doesn't require "damage control" by dieting or "escape" with alcohol or addictions. A big part of that is energy work and setting boundaries.

  - Boundaries. Much of our emotional stress comes from not saying no to things. We can't just get rid of stress, but we can decide that we can say no to things that drain us of good energy.

  - Mindful breathing/pranayama to balance the ANS. When you slouch in a chair or over a keyboard, your chest and heart are not expanded but concave. When you are stressed, your breathing is shallow. Did you ever wonder why you "sigh" heavily when you are stressed? Stress is metabolically demanding and saps you of crucially needed oxygen, pushing you into an anaerobic state; that's why you sigh heavily to resuscitate your increasingly oxygen-deprived cells. If you are not breathing into all lobes of your lungs, you are mildly asphyxiating yourself. When I used to teach yoga, I invited people to be mindful of their breath, both on and off the mat. I would say, "We can live weeks without food, days without water, but only a few minutes without air." Give your cells the gift of oxygen. Stand tall, lengthening your spine, energizing your shoulder blades down towards your tailbone. This posture allows more air to oxygenate your blood and cells. The easiest breath you can do to balance your ANS is to focus on having a longer exhale than inhale and then holding the exhale before inhaling.

Three of my favorite mindful breathing techniques for relaxation are:

- Ujjayi breath/ocean breath. By focusing on making your breath audible, you calm your mind while energizing your body. These breaths are done through the nose with the lips closed. Slightly constrict the back of your throat so that your air becomes audible, sort of like you saying *haaaaaa* to fog a mirror. Once you get the hang of it on the exhale, continue on to achieve the audible breath on the inhale as well.
- Box breathing. This is a good breathing technique for beginners as it only requires deep breathing and counting. It helps induce relaxation while reducing anxiety. Inhale through the nose for a count of four, hold the breath for a count of four, exhale for a count of four, and hold for a count of four. Doing this only three or four times is enough to notice more calmness. This breath can be enhanced by keeping the tip of the tongue gently pressing the area above the back of your upper front teeth.
- Alternate nostril breathing/Nadi Shodhana – This one is almost intoxicating because it streamlines oxygen right into the brain! It is somehow simultaneously grounding, centering, and energizing. I use this when I am nervous, like before public speaking, and when I need to stay awake, like when driving late at night. But the weird thing is, it can also help you to fall asleep! Again, there are a ton of blogs and videos that demonstrate this technique, but it is essentially closing off one nostril at a time for each inhalation/exhalation cycle.
- EMFs. All right, this one might sound a little "conspiracy theory" or "woo-woo" to some folks, but the research is rapidly accumulating for this, which is why entire cities are starting to ban 5G. I can't speak about this quite as eloquently as lots of other practitioners can, but I do know that the scientific papers are out there; you just have to seek out this information. If you have any doubts about this at all, this one is, at the very least, a "definitely might help, can't hurt" tip to try. Other countries seem to take more precautions than we do in the US. For instance, China strongly encourages pregnant women to wear EMF-protective aprons while France banned Wi-Fi in nursery schools in 2014. Israel requires warnings on all cell phones that state, "Warning – the Health Ministry cautions that heavy use and carrying the device next to the body may

increase the risk of cancer, especially among children." Israel also mandates that all cell phone ads reflect these warnings and bans cell phone advertisements directed towards children. Children are much more susceptible to the effects of radiation than adults because their tissues are still developing. And even cell phone manuals in the US say not to place it within an inch of our heads! Switch your phone to airplane mode any time you are not actively using it. This will not only cut down on the radiation you will be exposed to, but it can help break the habit of constantly looking at your phone for a dopamine hit in the event that someone messages you. Even if you are switching out of airplane mode once every 15 minutes, that's a considerable amount less radiation that's firing away at your cells each day. Try to keep your devices at least a foot away from your body. At the very least, put them in the outermost pocket of your bag or purse. Consider using air tube earbuds to keep radiation from your phone farther away from your head. Studies show that cellular damage is in direct proportion to the proximity of devices to the body. The "inverse-square law" specifies that intensity is inversely proportional to the square of the distance from the source of radiation (Miller et al. 2019). Use the speaker if earbuds are not an option at the time.

o Consider hardwiring your devices. At the very least, turn your router off at night (Christmas light timers are great!) or, better yet, when not in use. It's a bonus if you can move your router to a less commonly used area of your home. Again, wireless damage is in direct proportion to the distance between the body and the device.

o Supplement with magnesium. Now, I don't know if you have a favorite mineral, but I do, and it's magnesium. It was my favorite before I even learned that supplementing with it can help to reduce the harmful effects of EMFs. EMFs activate voltage-gated calcium channels, which are in the membranes of cells, allowing calcium to flow into the cell. Since magnesium is a natural calcium antagonist, it works as a calcium channel blocker (Houston 2011). In addition to this, magnesium participates in a vast number of other processes in the body, so supplementing with it has plenty of other health-promoting benefits.

o Selenium. Research in rats demonstrates that electromagnetic radiation can have a detrimental impact on the male reproductive system (Bilgici et al. 2018). Moreover, research demonstrates that EMF damage can be prevented by use of selenium (Khoshbakht et al. 2021). Ensure you are getting enough selenium but not too much, as it is toxic at high doses. The government has set the "tolerable upper intake level" at 400 micrograms (mcg). The RDA for selenium for people age 14 and older is 55 mcg and more during pregnancy and lactation.

Selenium is fairly common in foods, with Brazil nuts having the highest content. Be careful not to overconsume Brazil nuts, which can happen very easily – you only need a few.

○ Body movement. While certain types of exercise can help or hinder your wellness progression, your current biophysical state will determine which form will best suit your goals. In other words, while some forms of exercise may have proven benefits and make you feel good immediately afterwards, they may be too much for someone struggling with weak adrenal regulation, causing a hardcore need for a nap two hours later or else it creates inflammation and the inability to trim down or to get pregnant.

○ Exercise encourages lymph flow, circulation, and oxygenation in the body. This helps detox hormones, strengthen muscles, and reduce stress, as well as many other benefits. Exercise doesn't have to be high intensity but just regular, moderate body movement like my personal fun favorites, bicycling and roller skating.

○ Unlike the circulatory system, the lymphatic system does not have a pump, so body movement is absolutely necessary. The lymphatic system depends on the relaxation and contraction of muscles and joints to keep it moving; otherwise, it will get sluggish.

○ Regarding fertility, moving the lymphatic fluids helps boost immune system functioning and clear toxins, biological waste, and various types of proteins, including hormones. If toxins and waste are not cleared (called "autointoxication"), inflammation will ensue, which causes oxidative stress, which is at the root of impaired fertility.

○ Walking. It's good for everyone! Find your pace and distance.

○ Yoga. Since it has been practiced for thousands of years, there's gotta be something to it that gives it its staying power. It turns out that there are many benefits. Yoga can be a great way to stretch and loosen muscles. It gets the heart pumping. It balances the autonomic nervous system (fight/flight versus rest/digest/reproduce). It promotes GABA (a calming neurotransmitter). There are a plethora of types and intensities of yoga, so experiment with different styles or switch it up from time to time.

○ Qigong boosts immune response by improving lymph flow throughout the body. Since it focuses on breath, as does yoga, it helps oxygenate the cells. Being a form of "meditation in motion," it helps decrease stress. I personally find that it helps me have a more even, present mood throughout the day.

• Be sure to address lymphatic drainage prior to/at the beginning of any detox protocol. Some other ways to stimulate lymph drainage are jumping/bouncing on a rebounder, dry brushing, castor oil packs, and simply bouncing on an exercise ball. Movement is king, and gadgets/modalities are adjunct.

- Improve vagal tone. Many of these action steps also benefit the body by strengthening the vagus nerve to improve "vagal tone." The vagus nerve is a primary part of the parasympathetic nervous system (PNS) that regulates involuntary bodily functions and stimulates the "rest, digest, repair, and reproduce digest" (also called "feed and breed") states that occur when the body is at rest and stress-free.
  - The vagus nerve is often referred to as the "superhighway that connects the brain to the gut/microbiome and internal organs (and vice versa)." It runs messages anywhere to/from the brain all the way from/to the cervix and regulates nearly every major organ in between, including heart, lungs, esophagus, intestines, and reproductive organs. When the vagus nerve is stimulated, the PNS is soothed, calming the body and causing blood pressure and heart rate to lower. Digestion also improves when we are in this state.
  - Stimulating the vagus nerve to improve vagal tone has been shown to provide numerous health benefits. In fact, the FDA has approved vagus nerve stimulation for therapeutic use in chronic inflammatory and autoimmune conditions due to its anti-inflammatory properties (Johnson and Wilson 2018). Because of its important involvement throughout the entire body, whole books have been written on this underrepresented topic. Here area few basic, inexpensive methods to improve vagal tone.
  - Action steps here are some easy ways to stimulate the vagus nerve:
    - Gargle several times a day. Do it vigorously until your eyes water. Gargling contracts muscles in the back of the throat, which activates the vagus nerve. Put a sticky note on your mirror by your toothbrush to remind yourself to get into this habit.
    - Sing or hum loudly. Again, this activates the muscles in the back of the throat.
    - Deep breathing techniques, including yoga and chanting "om" causes vibration around the ear, where branches of the vagus nerve run through.
    - Cold exposure. Anything from cryotherapy to splashing cold water on your face. One practice that you can ease into is ending your shower by turning the faucet to the coldest setting before getting out. Ideally, work your way up to a full three minutes or longer. Even if you have to start with three seconds, that will still provide benefits and is better than not doing the cold water at all.

ACTION STEPS

- Acknowledge and address emotional traumas and blockages. Even though a lot of people discount or disregard this point, emotional traumas are finally getting the recognition they need when it comes to health and wellness. I want to move the conversation further and include emotional traumas as stressors that can impact fertility issues. Even though an emotional stressor may have happened many years ago, the imprint it leaves on the nervous system (and, eventually, the physical body) can last a literal lifetime unless consciously addressed. Emotional traumas are stressful to the point of being unconscious but potent stressors. Our bodies hold emotional scars that block energetic flow in the body, just like a physical scar does.

- Emotional trauma, inducing consequences of excessive stress/distress, not only blocks energetic flow but can also lead to greater health maladies later in life. Here's the science: Adverse childhood experiences, or ACEs, are potentially traumatic events that occur in childhood. ACEs are, unfortunately, all too common. According to the CDC, about 61% of adults surveyed across 25 states reported that they had experienced at least one type of ACE, and nearly one in six reported they had experienced four or more types of ACEs.

- ACEs have been shown to affect health outcomes, including fertility. A paper entitled "Adverse childhood event experiences, fertility difficulties and menstrual cycle characteristics" (Jacobs et al. 2015) states that child traumatic stress has been associated with neuroendocrine disruptions, including altered functioning of the hypothalamic-pituitary-adrenal (HPA) axis and raising cortisol levels.

- And don't think this just starts after you're born. There are many studies showing that babies absorb cortisol through the placenta (Murphy 1979), which can impact their nervous system and HPA axis/hormone control center. Fetal exposure to superabundant glucocorticoids can result in lifelong effects on neuroendocrine function (Whirledge and Cidlowski 2010). This is one reason I am a big believer in having the most natural, blissful birth you can because we are the same physical and emotional beings that we were since before birth, and many births these days are just as traumatic for the baby as they are for the mom. For anyone who will be giving birth, I strongly suggest hiring a doula. Having a doula at your labor and birth usually results in a more positive birth experience. Doulas offer comfort measures, education, advocacy, and physical and emotional support for both the birthing mother and her partner. Studies show that having a doula results in a shortened hospital stay with fewer interventions during the birthing process (Kennell et al. 1991; Harris et al. 2012).

- It's not just in utero, either. Stress-induced levels of glucocorticoids (steroidal hormones that are produced by the body in response to stress) have been shown to impair oocyte competence (Joseph and Whirledge 2017). What this means is that stress affects egg quality (Prasad et al. 2016).

- This also applies to men. As touched on in Chapter 2, fathers play a larger role in reproductive outcomes than most people assume. There are quite a few articles discussing findings that poor diet, lifestyle, and trauma create epigenetic changes in sperm. Men can pass on traumas epigenetically through sperm.

- Additionally, if the parent has unresolved trauma (even transgenerational trauma), then that can affect how that person parents, affecting the potential for ACEs even further.
- Mental and emotional dis-ease can lead to physical disease. In the same way that anxiety creates a racing heart or sweaty hands in the short term, other emotions can create short- or long-term physical manifestations. Emotional trauma is not limited to extremely negative events. It can be something as seemingly simple as a parent who didn't acknowledge you when arriving home from work every day or a single, deep-cutting comment. It can stem from anything that makes you feel dis-ease or uneasy. This can be small, repeated occurrences or a one-time event. Either way, it is something that is carried with you, consciously or not. There are a surprisingly high number of therapies and modalities that can help people work through emotional traumas. A fantastic place to start is at Inaura.com. Inaura is an interactive platform that helps you find resources to support your healing, growth, and self-discovery journey. It features high-quality education, world-class professional guides, classes, workshops, and much more – across the full spectrum of mental, emotional, and spiritual well-being. Refer to the resources section for more information.
- Chiropractic and/or craniosacral therapy. If energy is blocked, whether by physical injury or emotional injury, it will not flow or allow the flow of fluids as readily. Craniosacral therapy is a therapy that uses gentle touch to detect physical and emotional blockages and/or imbalances within the body and helps bring them into balance. My craniosacral therapist is mind-blowingly amazing. One example of why I know this is because, at the end of one of our sessions, she asked me if I'd had any root canals or major dental work, to which I told her I had gotten a mercury filling removed in Mexico about 12 years prior (and not by a biological dentist), and she said, "On the top left?" I had been wearing a face mask due to COVID requirements, and my mind was blown that she could pick up on that! She said she could tell that my immune system was reacting to it. Additionally, I always feel so symmetrical, grounded, and *open* when I get off her table. There is a whole gray-scale of modalities and practitioner talent, but try a few out, and I'm sure you'll find a modality and a practitioner match. I like my chiropractor and will likely stick with her as long as I can, but I had been to quite a few other chiropractors before finding her.
- Tapping, also referred to as the emotional freedom technique (EFT), is my favorite "might help, can't hurt" therapy, especially because I have found it to be a tremendous help. Sarah Holland and Naomi Woolfson are fertility practitioners in the UK who specialize in EFT.

REFERENCES

Bilgici, Birşen, Seda Gun, Bahattin Avci, Ayşegül Akar, and Begüm K. Engiz. 2018. "What is adverse effect of wireless local area network, using 2.45 GHz, on the reproductive system?" *International Journal of Radiation Biology* 94, no. 11, 1054–1061.

Harris, Susan J., Patricia A. Janssen, Lee Saxell, Elaine A. Carty, George S. MacRae, and Karen L. Petersen. 2012. "Effect of a collaborative interdisciplinary maternity care program on perinatal outcomes." *CMAJ* 184, no. 17, 1885–1892.

Houston, Mark. 2011. "The role of magnesium in hypertension and cardiovascular disease." *The Journal of Clinical Hypertension* 13, no. 11, 843–847.

Jacobs, Marni B., Renee D. Boynton-Jarrett, and Emily W. Harville. 2015. "Adverse childhood event experiences, fertility difficulties and menstrual cycle characteristics." *Journal of Psychosomatic Obstetrics & Gynecology* 36, no. 2, 46–57.

Johnson, Rhaya L., and Christopher G. Wilson. 2018. "A review of vagus nerve stimulation as a therapeutic intervention." *Journal of Inflammation Research* 11, 203.

Joseph, Dana N., and Shannon Whirledge. 2017. "Stress and the HPA axis: balancing homeostasis and fertility." *International Journal of Molecular Sciences* 18, no. 10, 2224.

Kennell, John, Marshall Klaus, Susan McGrath, Steven Robertson, and Clark Hinkley. 1991. "Continuous emotional support during labor in a US hospital: a randomized controlled trial." *Jama* 265, no. 17, 2197–2201.

Khoshbakht, Sareh, Fatemeh Motejaded, Sareh Karimi, Narjes Jalilvand, and Alireza Ebrahimzadeh-Bideskan. 2021. "Protective effects of selenium on electromagnetic field-induced apoptosis, aromatase P450 activity, and leptin receptor expression in rat testis." *Iranian Journal of Basic Medical Sciences* 24, no. 3, 322.

Miller, Anthony B., Margaret E. Sears, L. Lloyd Morgan, Devra L. Davis, Lennart Hardell, Mark Oremus, and Colin L. Soskolne. 2019. "Risks to health and well-being from radio-frequency radiation emitted by cell phones and other wireless devices." *Frontiers in Public Health* 223.

Murphy, Beverley E. Pearson. 1979. "Cortisol and cortisone in human fetal development." *Journal of Steroid Biochemistry* 11, no. 1, 509–513.

Oschman, James L., Gaétan Chevalier, and Richard Brown. 2015. "The effects of grounding (earthing) on inflammation, the immune response, wound healing, and prevention and treatment of chronic inflammatory and autoimmune diseases." *Journal of Inflammation Research* 8, 83.

Prasad, Shilpa, Meenakshi Tiwari, Ashutosh N. Pandey, Tulsidas G. Shrivastav, and Shail K. Chaube. 2016. "Impact of stress on oocyte quality and reproductive outcome." *Journal of Biomedical Science* 23, no. 1–5.

Sansone, Randy A., and Lori A. Sansone. 2013. "Sunshine, serotonin, and skin: A partial explanation for seasonal patterns in psychopathology?" *Innovations in Clinical Neuroscience* 10, no. 7–8, 20.

Whirledge, Shannon, and John A. Cidlowski. 2010. "Glucocorticoids, stress, and fertility." *Minerva endocrinologica* 35, no. 2, 109.

7 Mold and Mycotoxins: Get the Mold Out

Mold has been around for millions of years. Its role in the ecosystem is important in that it facilitates the decomposition of organic matter. There are many species of mold that are not harmful to our bodies and some that are even beneficial, but some produce toxins that are very detrimental to our health.

It seems only in recent years that mold toxicity has become quite an issue for many people. Our immune systems are constantly on high alert these days (as opposed to preindustrial days), coupled with a liver burden that "gums up" the removal of toxins and biotoxins (toxins produced by living organisms) like mold. Many people are not aware of their exposure to mold (and its cronies that exacerbate it) because much of it is not macroscopically visible.

Molds produce toxins called mycotoxins when they are disturbed or feel threatened. They do this as a way to protect themselves and the area around them from other molds intruding on their space. This is why they are more toxic and problematic than molds found outdoors, where there is more space for them to not feel threatened. Mold readily proliferates in warm, humid, damp places. Molds themselves aren't usually harmful, but the mycotoxins they produce are. Mycotoxins are any toxic substance produced by a fungus and are well documented for their toxic effects on human cells. Because they are tiny and fat soluble, mycotoxins can get into cell membranes and mitochondria and cause disruptions. Most known mycotoxins are cytotoxic (i.e., they're toxic to your cells), disrupting cellular structures and decreasing cellular energy production (ATP) by downregulating cellular function. We need cellular energy for reproduction!

Mycotoxins can be toxic to humans, animals, and the microorganisms around them. While they can be found almost anywhere mold is, mycotoxins are estimated to affect 25% of the world's crops (2018), including grains (especially corn), nuts, wine, spices, and coffee. This can be due to poor harvesting practices, improper food storage, or damp conditions during food transport and processing. Routes of exposure include absorption through the skin, inhalation (common with exposure to mold from water-damaged buildings), and when they are produced by mold in the GI tract or other organs (International College of Integrative Medicine 2019).

Mold can bioaccumulate if the body cannot effectively and quickly clear it. Even if you haven't been regularly exposed recently, the mold from your childhood house or college dorm can be affecting you today. Vulnerability to and symptomatology (i.e., the set of symptoms) of mycotoxins depends on the amount and duration of the exposure, genetic predisposition, age, health, and sex, as well as dietary status and interactions with other toxic insults.

DOI: 10.1201/b23201-9

An article in *Clinical Microbiology Reviews* states this information, as well as the following:

> The severity of mycotoxin poisoning can be compounded by factors such as vitamin defi-
> ciency, caloric deprivation, alcohol abuse, and infectious disease status. In turn, myco-
> toxicosis (i.e., system poisoning by mycotoxins) can heighten vulnerability to microbial
> diseases, worsen the effects of malnutrition, and interact synergistically with other toxins.
> (Bennett and Klich 2003)

This perfectly explains why there can be numerous people inhabiting a moldy building, and some people are riddled with symptoms, and others aren't noticing anything. People who are immunocompromised will generally be more affected; however, if exposure is prolonged or cumulative, it's only a matter of time until symptoms start popping up.

Because it affects numerous systems within the body, mold illness can present in a vast array of symptoms, so it can be hard to diagnose. Some common symptoms are:

- Chronic sinus and upper respiratory issues
- Chronic fatigue
- Chronic headaches
- Hormone imbalances
- Hypothyroid
- Fibromyalgia
- Foggy thinking
- Weight gain/weight loss resistance
- Neurological issues
- Joint pain
- Skin issues
- Multiple chemical sensitivities and histamine intolerance
- Anxiety
- Depression
- Frequent urination
- Sleep issues
- Reproductive issues
- Gut/digestive issues and distress

The tricky part is that mold toxicity mimics many of these conditions, so it can be really hard to tease apart.

Let's meet a few of the common molds and/or the mycotoxins they produce:

- *Penicillium* is a common mold genus that often grows in indoor environments and produces a wide range of mycotoxins. It is frequently encountered in water-damaged buildings. Carpet, wallpaper, fiberglass insulation,
  and soft furniture are the big culprits. *Penicillium* also commonly grows on
  citrus fruits and grains.

- Mycophenolic acid is a mycotoxin produced by the *Penicillium* fungus and has been well documented to be associated with miscarriage. Mycophenolic is profoundly immunosuppressive. In fact, it is used to make immunosuppressive drugs! The glucuronidation pathway is the phase 2 liver detox pathway that clears mycophenolic acid. Having SNPs in genes related to the glucuronidation pathway, especially the UGT1A10 gene (Mojarrabi and Mackenzie 1997), may inhibit mycophenolic acid clearance. I detail this pathway in Chapter 13.
- Aflatoxins are produced by a couple of different *Aspergillus* species. There are multiple types of aflatoxins, with aflatoxin B1 being one of the most toxic and carcinogenic. Aflatoxins are often associated with peanut products and are also found in milk from cows fed with contaminated grain. Aflatoxin B1 is also found in cottonseed oil. Aflatoxin and ochratoxin, as far as research currently shows, are only cleared by the phase 2 liver detox pathway of glutathione conjugation. The two most significant (and relatively common) genetic variants that can affect clearance of these two mycotoxins are GSTA and GSTM (Deng et al. 2018). These genes are also integral in detoxifying estrogen, so variants here will hinder estrogen clearance as well. The phase 1 liver detox gene, CYP3A4, metabolizes 98% of aflatoxin B1 (Yamada et al. 2020). Aflatoxin B1 is the most potent carcinogen that is metabolized by cytochrome P450 (CYP450) (Khan et al. 2021).
- Ochratoxin A is produced by *Aspergillus* and various species of *Penicillium* and, again, is commonly found in buildings that have had water damage. Phase 1 detox gets severely inhibited when Ochratoxin A is present. The kidneys and liver are most vulnerable to this toxin (Xia et al. 2021). Aside from potential issues to our own livers, we should keep this in mind when eating animal liver as well. Be sure to eat high-quality, grass-fed animal products, as feed grains are commonly contaminated. This mycotoxin has been shown to cause fetal death in animals (Still et al. 1971). Supporting the Nrf2 pathway, especially the NFE2L2 and KEAP1 genes, can help to keep this toxin from wreaking havoc. Refer to Appendix 11 for more information on these genes.
- Zearalenone (ZEA) mycotoxin is produced by certain types of *Fusarium* mold and is estrogenic in that it is an estrogen-mimicker; it can bind to estrogen receptors and has been shown in animal studies to be a reproductive toxin. It is cleared via the phase 2 liver detox pathways of glucuronidation and methylation. Zearalenone down-regulates immune response, leaving us more vulnerable to harmful pathogens. Again, this is a toxin commonly found in grains. Studies on various species of animals have shown that zearalenone can decrease fertility in males and females. Researchers have shown that exposure to ZEA can negatively affect ovulatory cycles (Smith et al. 1990), likely caused by the negative feedback loop that the estrogenic properties ZEA has on the pituitary gland. ZEA also affects oocyte maturation, can cause chromosomal mutations in those that do mature (Minervini et al. 2001), and increases deformities of male genitals and skeletal and soft

tissue in fetuses (Becci et al. 1982). Additionally, ZEA's estrogenic properties, coupled with how mycotoxins can bioaccumulate in the body, may lead
to estrogenic cancers from long-term exposure.

- Trichothecenes are produced by Stachybotrys ("black mold") and *Fusarium*,
among other molds, and commonly proliferate in water-damaged buildings.
They also frequently contaminate grain crops, causing poisoning in animals
eating contaminated feed (wheat, corn, oats, rye, barley). This toxin can affect
us when we consume the meat, eggs, and dairy products from animals that
are fed contaminated grains. In fact, eating trichothecene-contaminated animal products is the primary cause of human poisoning (Janik et al. 2021).
Stachybotrys is a "sticky" mold, so it often does not show up in air sample testing. Trichothecenes are very, very toxic to humans in acute or chronic exposures. Studies have shown trichothecenes, specifically T-2 toxin, to disturb the
hypothalamic, pituitary, and ovarian axis and also reduce sperm production
(and morphology) and serum testosterone concentration (Janik et al. 2021).

Although there are over 300 known mycotoxins, trichothecenes, fumonisins, ochra-
toxins, and aflatoxins are the most commonly encountered.

7.1 MOLD SPORES

Molds release tiny spores (invisible to the naked eye) in an attempt to propagate.
Spores enter our homes in various ways, including open windows and doors, vents,
and when they are brushed against, and they often hitch a ride inside buildings on
pets and clothing. Spores are common in our homes and don't become problematic unless they are able to germinate and become mold in the presence of moisture
and organic matter. Spores can spread and even survive for years in the absence of
moisture. Unfortunately, some of the places that tend to be great mediums for mold
growth are drywall, wood, concrete, ceiling tiles, carpets, mattresses, and upholstery.
If there have been any leaks, floods, or dampness from humidity or condensation,
mold would be able to thrive – and in as little as two to three days. This includes leaks
from appliances. Mold spores themselves are not toxic like mycotoxins, but they can
cause allergic reactions like sneezing and wheezing.

7.2 MYCOTOXINS AND GUT HEALTH

When we ingest food contaminated with mycotoxins, our intestinal barrier function,
nutrient absorption, and microbiome can be affected. This ultimately can (and likely
will) damage intestinal villi, which are finger-like projections in the intestinal lining
that are responsible for the absorption of fluids and nutrients. If we can't absorb nutrients, we will become malnourished and not have the nutrient reserves to grow a baby.
Also, intestinal microvilli are what produce the histamine-degrading enzyme diamine
oxidase (DAO) that I detail in Chapter 15 on histamine. If the villi are damaged, then
less DAO will be produced, leading to histamine intolerance and inflammation.

    When mycotoxins disrupt the microbiota, they create dysbiosis, which is when there
is an imbalance of good gut bacteria in relation to bad bacteria. This impairs the body's

ability to fight off harmful microbes, allowing them not only to set up shop in the body but also to weaken the immune system. We need to have an abundant amount and variety of beneficial bacteria residing in the gut to help aid in the mycotoxin removal process.

7.3 MOLD, MYCOTOXINS, AND REPRODUCTIVE HEALTH

Toxic mold exposure affects many systems of the body. It can disrupt mitochondrial function, thyroid hormones, sex and stress hormones, histamine regulation, and immune regulation. It also affects the limbic system, causing it to stay in "fight or flight" mode, which affects the nervous system and brain function.

Studies show that mycotoxins can cause cytotoxicity (destruction of cells, especially disrupting RNA and DNA synthesis), carcinogenicity (cancer generation), teratogenicity (agents that can disturb the development of the embryo or fetus), hepatotoxicity (liver toxicity), nephrotoxicity (toxicity to kidneys), neurotoxicity, and immunosuppression (Agriopoulou et al. 2020). They also can create autoimmune issues and wake dormant viruses, like the Epstein-Barr virus (EBV). All these characteristics can affect fertility directly and/or indirectly.

The *World Mycotoxin Journal* (Eze 2018) states that it is well established that mycotoxin exposure can have adverse effects on reproductive health, resulting in poor reproductive potential. The most studied mycotoxin in relation to poor reproductive health in humans is aflatoxin, although fumonisins, trichothecenes, and zearalenone have also been reported to impair reproductive function and cause abnormal fetal development (Eze 2018). These mycotoxins are a few that are cleared through the glucuronidation pathway (that is also a primary clearance pathway for hormones), so ensuring good phase 2 liver detox of that pathway (learn all about this in Chapter 13), as well as the others, will really help stave off reproductive issues.

Studies using animal and cell models indicate that zearalenone, deoxynivalenol, ochratoxin A, and aflatoxin B1 can adversely affect fertility through damage to sex organs, gametes, and disruption of steroidogenesis, which is the creation of sex and stress hormones. These particular mycotoxins have been shown in animal studies to promote adverse effects on spermatozoa, Sertoli cell (involved in sperm production), and Leydig cell (involved in production of testosterone) function; oocyte maturation; and uterine and ovarian development and function, both in vivo and ex-vivo (Eze 2016). These mycotoxins may also induce oxidative stress that results in sperm DNA damage, and prolonged exposure can lead to reduced fertilization rates and lower embryo quality.

Additionally, mycotoxins can act as endocrine disruptors and cause impaired fertility by altering hormonal balance (Kowalska et al. 2016; Santos et al. 2013; Bucheli et al. 2005).

It is interesting to note that maternal exposure to fumonisins from high corn-based food consumption have been linked to neural tube defects (Missmer et al. 2006). Again, this goes to show that we can't blame everything on the MTHFR genetic variant.

Mold is a potent mast cell activator. It also trashes our detoxification ability and our glutathione levels more than anything else. It is common for people who have issues with mycotoxins to end up with mast cell issues like mast cell activation syndrome (MCAS).

Since this book is about how oxidative stress and inflammation affect reproductive capacities, I'll state that oxidative stress is now understood to be a "significant mechanism of illness from exposure to water-damaged buildings" (Hope 2013). The statistics on water-damaged buildings surprised me. According to research conducted by the Insurance Information Institute, 98% of US basements experience some type of water damage (Hancock et al. 2021). Other statistics state that approximately 50% of US homes are estimated to have water damage and mold (Mudarri and Fisk 2007), with that percentage rising to an alarming 85% in commercial buildings. Many of my clients had been fairly certain that they had not been exposed to mold, and most of them had testing that proved otherwise. Consider mold and its mycotoxins to be a very large rock to look under for fertility challenges or any chronic and/or puzzling symptoms.

Mycotoxins don't just affect fertility. If a woman gets pregnant, many of these mycotoxins (and a whole host of other toxins) can pass from the mother to the fetus through the placenta. And that is not where it ends. This maternal exposure can absolutely continue during breastfeeding. If a woman feels the need to continue with binders once she gets pregnant and/or is breastfeeding, a more gentle and safe binder that has often been used is chlorella.

The consequences of aflatoxin exposure in mothers, fetuses, and children are many, including anemia in pregnancy, low birth weight, interference with nutrient absorption, suppression of immune function, child growth retardation (and developmental delay disorder), and abnormal liver function (Eze 2018).

7.4 TESTING FOR MYCOTOXINS IN THE BODY

For many practitioners, urine has been the preferred method for mycotoxin analysis because most mycotoxins are excreted via urine once they have been metabolized. However, just as with any form of testing, mycotoxin excretion tests may not always reflect the whole picture. Many people are not doing a lot of provocation before testing (to pull toxins out of storage), so we need to think about what we are seeing and not seeing. What this means is that someone could have mycotoxin colonization in their body, but if they are not detoxifying and clearing it well, it won't be excreted. We see what comes out, but we don't know what is still in there. This is why we can't just rely on test results. We need to consider case history, whether there is ongoing or previous exposure, what genetic pathways may be playing a part, and/or how well the associated phase 2 pathways are working.

Different mycotoxins from mold are detoxified through different phase 2 detox pathways, which I go into great detail about in Chapter 13 on precision liver detoxification. Many practitioners are just simply recommending glutathione for mycotoxicosis, but what they do not know is that only a couple of mycotoxins are actually detoxified through this pathway. This is great if that happens to be the particular mycotoxin taking up residence in your body, but it won't do much if it is not. Knowing what type of mold and mycotoxins you are dealing with is very helpful in being able to get them out of the body. This is where testing can be of tremendous benefit. The urine organic acids test can be a great first step to see what might be hanging out in your body, as a general ballpark. But if you're really having issues, then a mycotoxin profile (like those through Great Plains, Vibrant Wellness, or RealTime Labs) is more specific and will allow you to detox with precision (Figure 7.1).

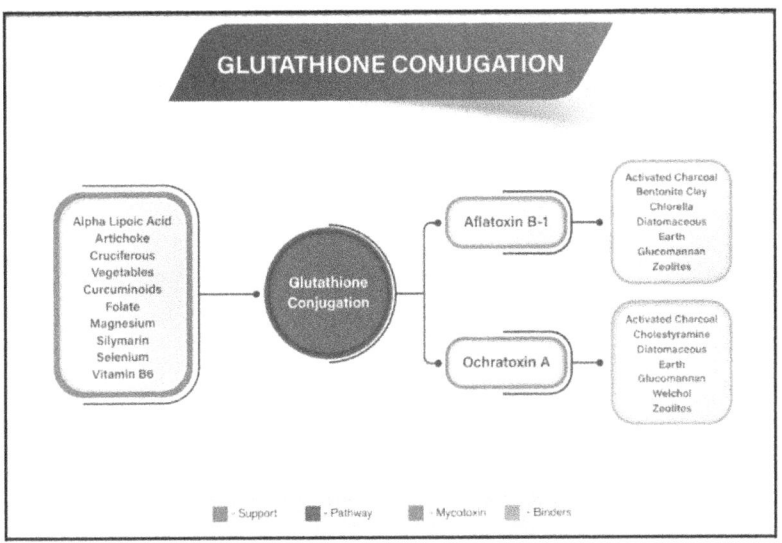

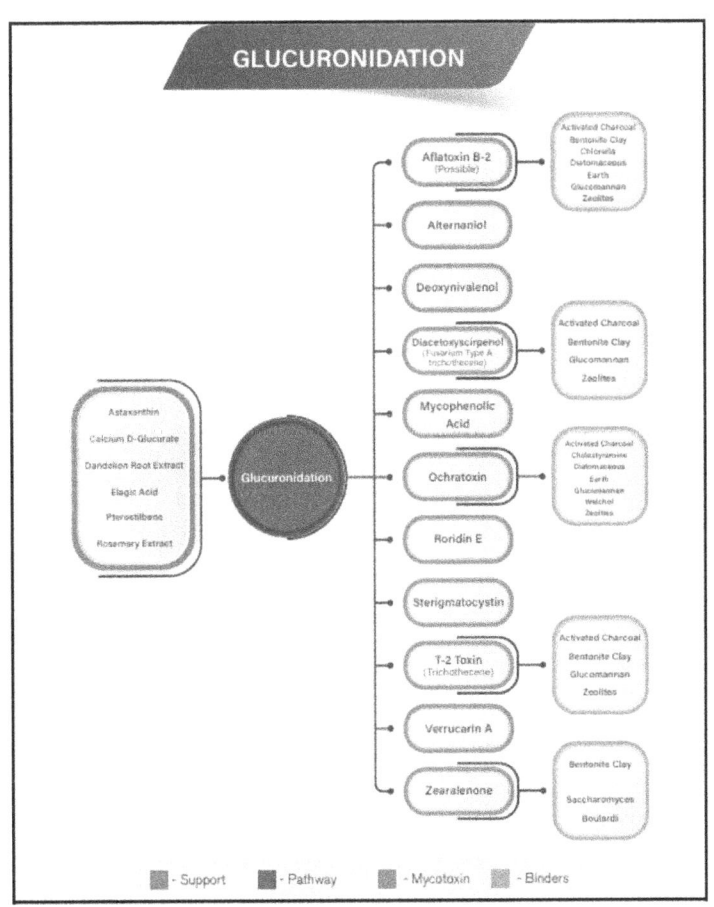

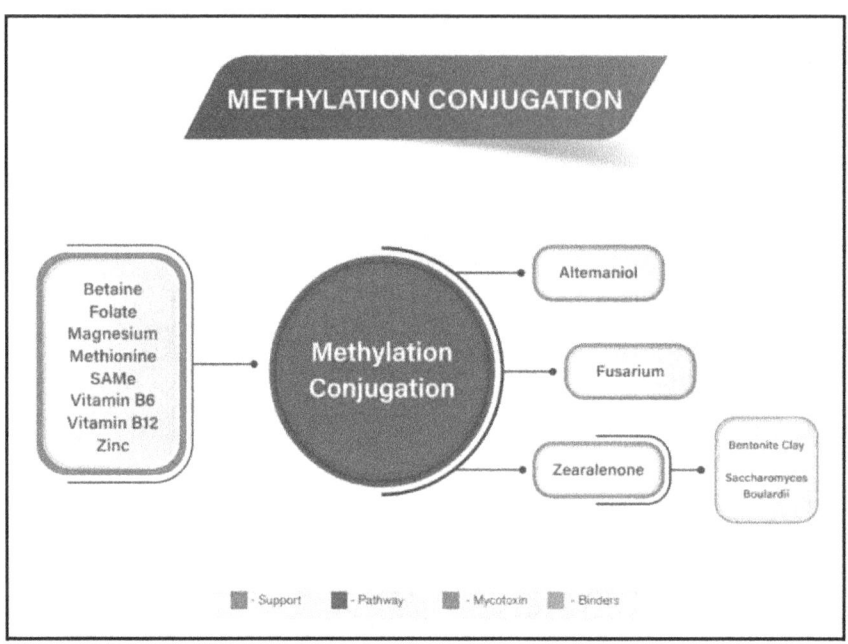

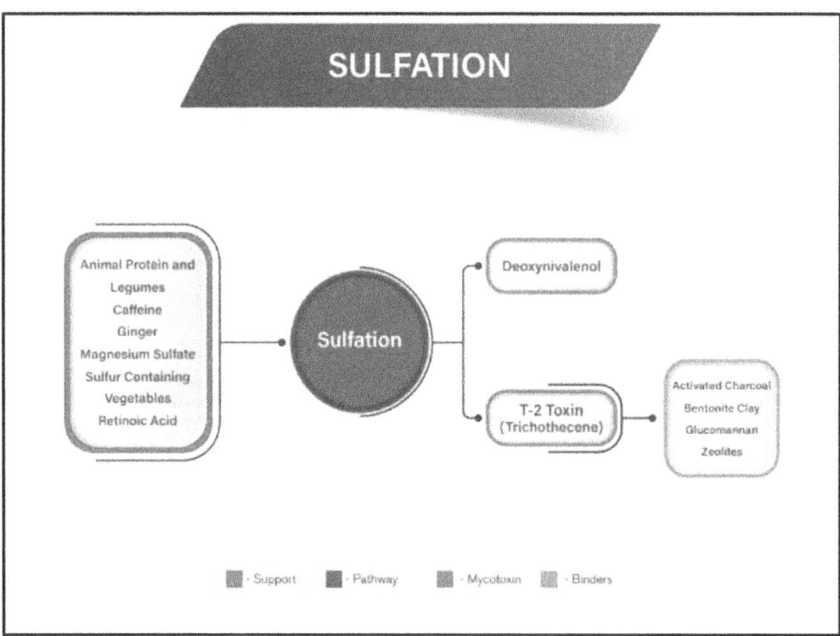

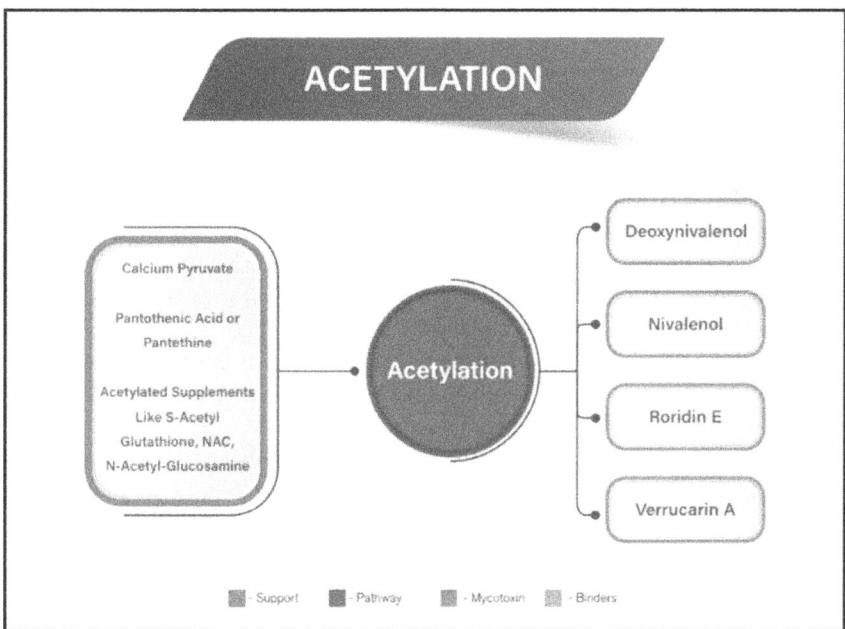

FIGURE 7.1 Nutrients, herbs, and foods that support each pathway, mycotoxins that are known to be cleared via each pathway, and the binders that are known to be effective for those mycotoxins.

Source: Reprinted with permission from Beyond Protocols: Comparison of mycotoxin detoxification by phase 2 liver detoxification pathways

Knowing which specific mycotoxins are causing issues in the body allows for precise interventions. Once we know this, we can know which phase 2 detoxification pathway(s) they are cleared through, and which herbs/nutrients/supplements upregulate that pathway. We also know which binders the research shows are most effective for specific types of mycotoxins.

There may be lots of layers compounding a situation, especially when it comes to impaired fertility. These layers can include emotional trauma, heavy metals, parasites, Lyme disease, coinfections, and the Herpes family viruses. Sometimes we need to open up a detox pathway to see what will show up in subsequent testing.

7.5 CLEARING OUT THE MOLD

As I mentioned, some mycotoxins can inhibit detoxification processes, so it is important to support/optimize these first before trying to detoxify specific substances. We are constantly exposed to various molds and mycotoxins. Our bodies have been designed to get rid of them, but when our detox pathways are overwhelmed, toxins will accumulate.

Action Steps

- First and foremost, if mycotoxins are present in your body, you must make sure you are not living or working in a moldy environment. Clearing mold from the body won't be much help if you continue to have ongoing exposure. Seek out a qualified mold inspector or building biologist. Refer to the resources section of this book.
- Balance the autonomic nervous system (ANS) – Get out of the sympathetic "fight or flight" response and into the parasympathetic healing mode (which the previous chapter detailed). Sympathetic nervous system dominance will allow stress to affect the liver and block the movement of bile. This will also cause enterohepatic recirculation, in which the toxins can't effectively get out of the body, so they get dumped back into the blood to be recirculated. This will only reinforce sympathetic dominance.
- Mold and mycotoxins affect so many parts of the body and can be very difficult to clear out. Balancing the autonomic nervous system is an important part of this process. Mindful breathing/pranayama, yoga, tai chi, meditation, qigong, getting serious about your sleep, and even just listening to binaural beats can help move you into a parasympathetic state so your body is more ready to detoxify, repair, and reproduce. See Chapter 6 for additional tips for balancing the ANS.
- Some herbs that are known for balancing the autonomic nervous system are Chinese skullcap (*Scutellaria baicalensis*), passionflower, and cannabinoids.
- The liver is the most important regulatory force in the body, especially when it comes to hormones. Hormonal harmony doesn't stand a chance if we don't have a properly working liver. If our liver and bile aren't working well, this will stress the adrenals, which leads to a whole host of hormone and HPA axis problems, including thyroid issues.
- Another easy way we can support and encourage the removal of toxins is to increase bile flow with bitters. Bitter herbs are known to aid digestion (especially of dietary fats) and stimulate bile flow that transports toxins from the liver to the intestines. Some common bitter herbs are dandelion root, burdock root, gentian root, and bitter green veggies like arugula and dandelion leaf.
- Binders will absolutely need to be in the lineup and are something I often recommend even before starting with targeted detoxification. I think of binders as a cleanup crew with lots of sponges. Binders will be the best friend of anyone who is trying to detoxify mold. Certain binders have affinities for certain mycotoxins. For instance, activated charcoal is great for aflatoxin B2 and ochratoxin, but bentonite clay and *Saccharomyces boulardii* are going to be more effective for zearalenone. Other binders that are commonly used for different types of mycotoxins are zeolite, glucomannan, and the prescription drugs Welchol and cholestyramine. This is where testing for mycotoxins in the body is super advantageous because you can get targeted precision with removal. Mold is hard on the systems in the body, so supporting the kidney, liver, and pituitary and adrenal glands is essential.

Even without any active detox support, people can take binders as a stand-alone, and they will still be effective at binding some degree of mycotoxins. As I mentioned a short bit ago, certain binders are more effective for some mycotoxins than others.

- Avoid alcohol. Alcohol pounds the immune system, feeds yeast, exacerbates intestinal permeability, wreaks havoc on hormones, disrupts sleep, and burdens the liver. Consider avoiding alcohol to be in every action step section written in this book!

- Bolster your antioxidant status since exposure to mold can stimulate the production of free radicals and inhibit endogenous antioxidant activity. This can be done through eating a wide variety of colorful foods that are rich in antioxidants (and juicing them), as well as through supplementation with things like resveratrol, vitamin C, vitamin E, and flavonoids.

- Nrf2, which modulates antioxidant response, is critical for the UGT enzyme function that drives glucuronidation. As I wrote in Chapter 13, astaxanthin can induce Nrf2 activity. Molecular hydrogen is a great way to support Nrf2 as well. In fact, molecular hydrogen is almost always in my protocols for people dealing with mold.

- Not all molds produce spores, but they always produce mycotoxins, so you need to test for mycotoxins, not just spores. This is why many functional medicine practitioners recommend an ERMI or EMMA test if someone suspects mold is an issue in their home, work environment, or any other place they spend a good amount of time. These are done by collecting samples onto a dust rag or something similar and sending it to the lab to be PCR tested. A second step to finding out where mold may be (including belongings/house items) is to order mold test plates from Immunolytics.[1] Aside from hiring a qualified and certified mold inspector or building biologist, these are usually the first steps I recommend for anyone who may live or work in an environment that smells musty, has had any degree of water damage (leaks, floods, larger spills), or has unexplainable symptoms that seem to have no cause. I would like to note that cars are surprisingly notorious for having mold, as are unfinished basements and crawl spaces.

- Consider urinary mycotoxin testing. When mold exposure has been prolonged or more abundant than the body can properly deal with, it can colonize in various areas of the body and wreak havoc. The caveat here is that if your liver is all clogged up and not working well, you won't be excreting toxins (including mycotoxins) very well, so doing follow-up urinary testing after supporting the liver can show much higher levels than an initial test. This is good! It means that your body is now getting rid of the gunk.

- Get sweaty! Many mycotoxins are lipophilic, which means they are attracted to and bind to the lipid portion of lipid proteins (i.e., lipoproteins). Because of this, mycotoxins can persist in the body for long periods of time (Wild and Gong 2010). Certain mycotoxins have been found in sweat, and sauna is often a useful therapy in helping people with mycotoxicosis to feel considerably better. Refer to the resources page for my favorite sauna recommendation and a special discount only offered for readers of this book.

- In addition to the gut, certain fungal infections commonly occur in the sinus cavities and lungs (e.g., pneumonia). Talk with your health practitioner about effective ways to clear out mold from these places, like nebulizing certain killing agents, for instance.
- Get the best air purifier you can afford and be diligent about using it with a clean filter.
- Use a dehumidifier. Humidity above 50–60% can lead to mold growth. I leave mine in my basement, set at 50% or lower at all times.
- Immediately clean up and dry out any water spills, leaks, or intrusions. Mold can start to grow as soon as 36 hours after initial exposure.
- Old house or new house – which is worse? Old houses, especially those with unfinished basements, are notorious for mold. However, many of my clients tell me they can't have mold issues because their house is new. The energy efficient houses today are built so much more tightly sealed than older houses. The houses today are also paper boxes that could have been exposed to rain during the building process. Do you think the builders wait until the house is adequately dried each time it rains? I don't. In some damp climates, that may never happen.
- Don't forget that your car can be a problem. If your windows were down when it rained, be sure to dry out floors and upholstery very well, and leave windows cracked when there is no chance of rain. Also, change the air filter regularly.
- Wash mold-exposed fabrics in borax. Borax is a natural mold and mildew killer that doesn't emit toxic fumes.
- *Do not use bleach*. I repeat, do not use bleach! Mold thrives in wet environments. Bleach is primarily water. Molds release mycotoxins as a defense mechanism when they feel stressed or threatened. If you bleach mold, it will kill the mold but release mycotoxins as a result and also create a wet space for more mold to potentially grow.
- As I stated, coffee is a common source of mycotoxins, so choose your brand carefully, or do some research to see if your brand has ever been tested for mycotoxins. Mycotoxins are often able to withstand high cooking temperatures, so the hot water in your coffee won't kill them.

NOTE

1   Test plates can be ordered through this link: https://immunolytics.com/?wpam_id=16.

REFERENCES

2018. www.ars.usda.gov/midwest-area/peoria-il/national-center-for-agricultural-utilization-research/mycotoxin-prevention-and-applied-microbiology-research/docs/what-are-mycotoxins/.
Agriopoulou, Sofia, Eygenia Stamatelopoulou, and Theodoros Varzakas. 2020. "Advances in occurrence, importance, and mycotoxin control strategies: prevention and detoxification in foods." *Foods* 9, no. 2, 137.

Becci, Peter J., William D. Johnson, Frederick G. Hess, Michael A. Gallo, Richard A. Parent, and Jean M. Taylor. 1982. "Combined two-generation reproduction-teratogenesis study of zearalenone in the rat." *Journal of Applied Toxicology* 2, no. 4, 201–206.

Bennett, J. W., and M. Klich. 2003. "Mycotoxins." *Clinical Microbiology Reviews* 497–516.

Bucheli, Thomas D., Marianne Erbs, Niccolo Hartmann, Susanne Vogelgsang, Felix E. Wettstein, and H. R. Forrer. 2005. "Estrogenic mycotoxins in the environment." *Mitteilungen aus Lebensmitteluntersuchung und Hygiene* 96, no. 6, 386.

Deng, Jiang, Ling Zhao, Ni-Ya Zhang, Niel Alexander Karrow, Christopher Steven Krumm, De-Sheng Qi, and Lv-Hui Sun. 2018. "Aflatoxin B1 metabolism: regulation by phase I and II metabolizing enzymes and chemoprotective agents." *Mutation Research/Reviews in Mutation Research* 778, 78–79.

Eze, U. A., S. E. M. Lewis, L. Connolly, and Y. Y. Gong. 2016. "Mycotoxins as potential cause of human infertility-a review of evidence from animal and cellular models." *III All Africa Horticultural Congress* 1225, 513–525.

Eze, U. A., M. N. Routledge, F. E. Okonofua, J. Huntriss, and Y. Y. Gong. 2018. "Mycotoxin exposure and adverse reproductive health outcomes in Africa: a review." *World Mycotoxin Journal* 11, no. 3, 321–339.

Hancock, Noah Scott, Shaheed H. Khan, and Kelvin J. Watson. 2021. "Proactive basement flood monitor." *ASEE North Central Section Conference.*

Hope, J. 2013. "Fungal contamination affects human olfactory systems with mycotoxins and allergens*: a review of the mechanism of injury and treatment approaches for illness resulting from exposure to water-damaged buildings, mold, and mycotoxins." *Scientific World Journal* 767482.

International College of Integrative Medicine. 2019. *Mycotoxins: Their effects on health and fertility.* https://icimed.com/mycotoxins-their-effects-on-health-and-fertility/.

Janik, Edyta, Marcin Niemcewicz, Marcin Podogrocki, Michal Ceremuga, Maksymilian Stela, and Michal Bijak. 2021. "T-2 toxin – the most toxic trichothecene mycotoxin: metabolism, toxicity, and decontamination strategies." *Molecules* 26, no. 22, 6868.

Khan, M. Tahir, M. Irfan, H. Ahsan, S. Ali, A. Malik, A. A. Pech-Cervantes, Z. Cui, Y. J. Zhang, and D. Q. Wei. 2021. "CYP1A2, 2A13, and 3A4 network and interaction with aflatoxin B1." *World Mycotoxin Journal* 14, no. 2, 179–189.

Kowalska, Karolina, Dominika Ewa Habrowska-Górczyńska, and Agnieszka Wanda Piastowska-Ciesielska. 2016. "Zearalenone as an endocrine disruptor in humans." *Environmental Toxicology and Pharmacology* 48, 141–149.

Minervini, F., M. E. Dell'Aquila, F. Maritato, P. Minoia, and A. Visconti. 2001. "Toxic effects of the mycotoxin zearalenone and its derivatives on in vitro maturation of bovine oocytes and 17β-estradiol levels in mural granulosa cell cultures." *Oxicology in Vitro* 15, no. 4–5, 489–495.

Missmer, Stacey A., Lucina Suarez, Marilyn Felkner, Elaine Wang, Alfred H. Merrill Jr, Kenneth J. Rothman, and Katherine A. Hendricks. 2006. "Exposure to fumonisins and the occurrence of neural tube defects along the Texas – Mexico border." *Environmental Health Perspectives* 114, no. 2, 237–241.

Mojarrabi, Behnaz, and Peter I. Mackenzie. 1997. "The human UDP glucuronosyltransferase, UGT1A10, glucuronidates mycophenolic acid." *Biochemical and Biophysical Research Communications* 238, no. 3, 775–778.

Mudarri, David, and William J. Fisk. 2007. "Public health and economic impact of dampness and mold." *Indoor Air* 17, no. LBNL-63007.

Santos, R. R., E. J. Schoevers, B. A. J. Roelen, and J. Fink-Gremmels. 2013. "Mycotoxins and female reproduction: in vitro approaches." *World Mycotoxin Journal* 6, no. 3, 245–253.

Smith, J. F., M. E. Di Menna, and L. T. McGowan. 1990. "Reproductive performance of Coopworth ewes following oral doses of zearalenone before and after mating." *Reproduction* 89, no. 1, 99–106.

Spengler, John, Lucas Neas, Satoshi Nakai, Douglas Dockery, Frank Speizer, James Ware, and Mark Raizenne. 1994. "Respiratory symptoms and housing characteristics." *Indoor Air* 4, no. 2, 78–82.

Still, P. E., A. W. Macklin, W. E. Ribelin, and E. B. Smalley. 1971. "Relationship of ochratoxin A to foetal death in laboratory and domestic animals." *Nature* 234, no. 5331, 563–564.

Wild, Christopher P., and Yun Yun Gong. 2010. "Mycotoxins and human disease: a largely ignored global health issue." *Carcinogenesis* 31, no. 1, 71–82.

Xia, Qing, Zhaolin Du, Dasong Lin, Lili Huo, Li Qin, Wei Wang, Liwen Qiang, Yanpo Yao, and Yi An. 2021. "Review on contaminants in edible oil and analytical technologies." *Oil Crop Science* 6, no. 1, 23–27.

Yamada, Marie, Koji Hatsuta, Mayuko Niikawa, and Hiromasa Imaishi. 2020. "Detoxification of aflatoxin B1 contaminated maize using human CYP3A4." *Journal of Microbiology and Biotechnology* 30, no. 8, 1207–1213.

8 Iron Behaving Badly: Understand Your Iron Status

An *incredibly* common root cause of inflammation is iron and copper dysregulation, which surprised me once it got on my radar!

I'd like to emphatically state that most available information about iron is antiquated and could be causing more harm than good. People blame MTHFR for their inflammation, but iron dysregulation is a *huge* contributing factor to the generation of free radicals that cause inflammation. When it comes to iron, people think that iron-deficiency anemia is most commonly the problem, when really, it is iron overload.

A large percentage of my clients, as well as clients of my colleagues, have a genetic predisposition for iron dysregulation, and blood testing often confirms that these genes are expressing and/or problematic. I'll be naming names (of genes) in this chapter so you will know what to look for on your genetic report.

But why is this so common?

In previous generations, holding on to iron was a genetic win for people in certain parts of the world because it kept people alive and even allowed women to carry pregnancies to term during famines. In recent decades, this has thankfully not been the case for the large majority of societies, so now holding on to excess iron can be detrimental to our health.

Iron is one of the most abundant minerals on earth. Even with that, fortification of foods with iron is commonplace. Unless someone has internal bleeding or a bleeding disorder (both termed hemorrhagic anemia) or has been on a strictly plant-based diet for quite some time, it's not likely that they have anemia from poor iron intake; it's likely an iron utilization issue.

Most doctors measure what's in the blood, which will look fine, or even low, because iron can be in excess *inside* the cells and tissues. Iron that is stuck inside the cell can't do its job and will oxidize, creating massive inflammation.

As that iron hangs around inside the cell, it creates fatigue because the mitochondria are having a hard time making energy (ATP).[1] As you will read repeatedly in this book, if the body isn't easily making energy, it knows it won't stand a chance of developing a baby.

I've seen it happen to people who were told to supplement with iron, and they felt considerably worse because they were feeding the fire; the iron was getting stuck in the wrong places and not able to go where it needed to.

DOI: 10.1201/b23201-10

Iron that is not able to be properly used will create free radicals through a process called the Fenton reaction. Refer to Appendix 8A for a deep dive into the Fenton reaction.

Improperly used iron will also feed viruses, bacteria, parasites, and fungi, including candida. This is one reason why some women are easily susceptible to yeast infections despite a low-carb diet and use of antifungals. You can get rid of candida, but if you don't change the terrain, there's still a ripe environment for it to be welcomed right back in.

What causes iron to be improperly used? Copper plays a *huge* part. If we don't have proper copper utilization, then our iron doesn't stand a chance. But then, you may be asking, what creates proper copper utilization?

Ceruloplasmin!

Refer to Appendix 8B for information about how copper and its binding protein, ceruloplasmin, are required for proper iron utilization and the related genes.

There are easy ways to increase your ceruloplasmin. Research in rats demonstrates that a major player involved in the synthesis of ceruloplasmin is retinol, the bioavailable form of vitamin A. The retinol is converted to retinoic acid and is a cofactor for the production of ceruloplasmin. However, retinol is only found in foods that come from animals, with the best sources being oily fish, liver, eggs, and cheese. Cod liver oil is a good food-based supplement for retinol.

Even though retinol is best known as being necessary for healthy eyes, teeth, hair, and skin and for immune system functioning, retinol is critical for fertility (Koricho et al. 2020) and reducing the severity of polycystic ovarian syndrome (PCOS) (Moayeri et al. 2020). It helps create healthy cervical fluid and follicle maturation and function, and it is also important for sperm health. Retinol regulates tissue differentiation so that cells know which organs to become, which is crucial in early fetal development.

What else helps make ceruloplasmin besides retinol/retinoic acid? Magnesium and copper. Yep, that's quite a catch 22, eh? We need ceruloplasmin to properly bind copper so that unbound/free copper won't create free radicals via the Fenton reaction, but we can't make ceruloplasmin without copper.

So many delicate dances that our amazing bodies host . . .

Copper, when it is properly used, plays a part in many functions in the body:

- It's essential for proper use of iron.
- It's required for energy production in the cells (if cells don't have proper energy production, they will shut down mating abilities).
- It is required for the copper form of superoxide dismutase (cu/zn SOD), an antioxidant.
- It assists in neurotransmitter production and regulation.
- It plays a big part in immune system functioning.
- It is important for cardiovascular system functioning.

A few common symptoms of copper deficiency are:

- Anemia (Remember that ceruloplasmin binds copper, and if we don't have enough of that, our iron utilization doesn't stand a chance.)

- Allergies/histamine intolerance (Copper helps degrade histamine.)
- Infertility
- Insomnia
- Anxiety
- Hypothyroidism

A few common symptoms of copper toxicity are:

- Physical and mental fatigue
- Poor memory
- Lack of concentration
- Inability to fall asleep and/or stay asleep
- Depression
- Sensitive temperament with extreme overreaction to events
- Headaches
- Cold extremities
- Nausea
- Vomiting
- Spaciness/brain fog
- Joint pain

Copper toxicity can damage the liver, kidneys, brain, and eyes. Symptoms of excess copper relating to fertility are reproductive issues, low libido, estrogen dominance, and the whole gamut of psychological problems that are rampant today. Again, that's just a tiny sample of symptoms.

A note on the copper IUD: Often preferred because it is not hormonal contraception, the copper IUD will continuously secrete micro doses of copper into the uterus for the purpose of creating an inflammatory effect that will damage and kill sperm. Consider the risk of copper toxicity before having a copper IUD inserted, especially if you are genetically prone to iron or copper dysregulation or zinc deficiency.

Because zinc and copper compete for the same absorption protein, metallothionein, when they are not in the proper ratio, zinc deficiency can cause copper toxicity. If you are going to supplement with one, you *must* be mindful of your levels of the other. I recommend keeping them in a ratio of about 10:1 zinc to copper, or not too far off from that. Proper testing in the form of a hair tissue mineral analysis (HTMA) and blood testing (measuring plasma zinc and serum copper, as well as ceruloplasmin) can tell you where the levels are in your blood and in storage and how much of each you need.

Although zinc and copper are antagonists, meaning they compete for absorption, they do work together. Together, they are well known for making the antioxidant enzyme superoxide dismutase, which is found in abundance in cells throughout the body.

Zinc is an incredibly important nutrient and is essential for hormone production (especially progesterone, our "pro-gestation" hormone), fertility, and miscarriage prevention, and a whole book could be written on its many uses in the body, but I don't want to stray too far off my initial point of needing copper for proper iron regulation.

8.1 WHILE HEMOCHROMATOSIS ISN'T ALL THAT COMMON, IRON DYSREGULATION IS

Hemochromatosis, also called "iron overload disorder," is a disorder that causes the body to absorb iron in excess amounts. Most people have not heard this term unless someone they know has it.

Because iron has a limited capacity to be excreted by the body, it can easily build up in joints and organs like the liver, heart, and pancreas; the GI tract; and even bone marrow. This is potentially problematic because iron is a potent oxidizer that can damage body tissues and can lead directly to lipid, protein, and DNA damage and ultimately cell death (Fraser et al. 2011). In extreme or long-term cases, iron overload has been linked to diabetes (Simcox and McClain 2013), cancer, heart disease, and retinal damage (Dunaief et al. 2014).

Refer to Appendix 8C for more information on various genes related to hemochromatosis and iron dysregulation.

Iron dysregulation isn't a black-or-white issue. People can still have tendencies to higher iron levels without having a genetic predisposition or a hemochromatosis diagnosis. This is much more likely to happen if you have missed periods or are on birth control that stops your periods.

A note for anemic women with heavy periods and/or more than one period per month: Your heavy periods may not be caused solely by hormone imbalance. They may be the result of iron dysregulation, in which the body is trying to get rid of excess iron. If you get on birth control to inhibit the body's compensatory mechanism of getting rid of excess iron (to lighten menstrual bleeding), this can become very problematic.

Studies have shown that hormonal imbalance is a significant problem for people with iron overload (Puntarulo 2005; O'Sullivan and Howel Walsh 2007). I mentioned earlier that iron can accumulate in the heart, brain, and other tissues, but it can also accumulate in the pituitary gland, which can disrupt the synthesis of gonadotropin-releasing hormone (GnRH), which stimulates the production of sex hormones from the ovaries and testes, creating abnormally low levels of estrogen and testosterone. This is something to consider if your estrogen is low, but your periods are heavy.

As I stated earlier, oftentimes, it is not an iron acquisition issue that is the problem; it is an iron utilization issue. If you have a predisposition to iron dysregulation, there are certain things you can do to improve iron utilization in the body, as well as dietary strategies to avoid absorbing too much iron. Just as people who have genetically related hemochromatosis often undergo medical bloodletting, donating blood is a great way to keep iron levels from becoming too high or iron depositing in organs. This is especially true for men and post-menopausal women.

Appendix 8D has information on reducing the Fenton reaction through reducing hydrogen peroxide.

Clearly, iron is an important mineral needed for many functions. However, if iron is in excess or it is not properly chaperoned through the body, it can become very dangerous, as iron is a potent oxidizer that can damage body tissues and cells.

Some causes of excess iron:

- Genetic predisposition
- Regular consumption of alcohol, as alcohol increases iron absorption
- Cooking in cast-iron skillets
- Iron fortification (This form is inorganic and can be much more dangerous than iron naturally occurring in foods.)
- Supplements containing iron
- Herpes and viral hepatitis (Mancinelli et al. 2020)

Dietary iron is a small part of our iron; 95% of our iron is recycled, and it may not be recycled properly. Lactoferrin and molecular hydrogen may help regulate this process.

Oxalates are an iron chelator, so anemia may be diagnosed if oxalates are a problem. Read more about oxalates in Chapter 9. If this is the case, you may see rust-colored crystals in the urine/feces as oxalates that are bound to iron are being shed.

ACTION STEPS

- Get a complete iron panel that includes more markers than just serum iron and hemoglobin. These are RBC magnesium, serum copper, zinc, ceruloplasmin, ferritin, and total iron-binding capacity (TIBC). It is also good to know your vitamin A status, if possible.

Here are a few nutritional products to improve the utilization and clearance of iron:

- Skullcap possesses antioxidant properties and is also antiviral. Studies in mice showed both quercetin and baicalin (an extract of skullcap) reduced iron-induced lipid peroxidation and protein oxidation in the liver, decreased liver iron stores as well as serum ferritin, and increased fecal excretion of iron (Zhang et al. 2006). Skullcap has many other uses, especially for reproductive and menstruation issues and nervous conditions.
- Lactoferrin modulates iron usage by binding to iron outside the bloodstream in areas like the GI tract and reproductive tissues (Jiang et al. 2011).
- Lipoic acid (R-lipoic acid is the most active form of alpha lipoic acid) is highly effective in reversing oxidative stress arising from iron overload, and its antioxidant efficacy is further enhanced in combination with acetyl-L-carnitine (Lal et al. 2008). Refer to Chapter 10 for info on carnitine.
- Phenolic-rich herbs and spices, like green tea and rosemary.

- Curcumin acts as an iron chelator to inhibit iron absorption. This may be one of the reasons it is such a great anti-inflammatory.
- Astaxanthin, which has many known health benefits, also reduces iron-induced oxidative damage.
- Some herbs and spices, like cloves, also inhibit iron absorption, as do tannins from various types of teas.
- Chlorophyll contains a porphyrin ring that can chelate up to 12 times its weight in toxic heavy metals and iron; let that be your reminder to eat plenty of greens!

Here are some tips that may help with iron, copper, and/or ceruloplasmin optimization.

- Unless you are pregnant or nursing or have a bleeding disorder, you may want to consider avoiding supplements and foods that have iron added. This is typically the unbound/free, non-heme iron, which fuels the Fenton reaction. I'm not saying to never take iron supplements, as I don't follow an "always/never" approach. This is where it is important to get comprehensive lab work to see the full picture and to have a doctor you feel comfortable talking to. I had a client who had ferritin in the low single digits, and the only thing that worked quickly enough to raise it was iron infusions.
- If you do have low ferritin or iron, there are things you can do to help support your levels while addressing the root cause of why you are low in the first place. Desiccated grass-fed liver capsules may be something to consider, as the liver is the heme form (bioavailable), and it also contains retinol to support ceruloplasmin, as well as being a cornucopia of B vitamins, choline, zinc, copper, and other trace minerals. Grass-fed, clean-sourced liver has a plethora of other health benefits as well.
- Avoid ascorbic acid forms of vitamin C. Since it doesn't contain the wide array of bioflavonoids, ascorbic acid is only a partial form of what you will find in food-based sources, and this form inhibits ceruloplasmin, which is needed for proper copper binding and iron utilization. Also, ascorbic acid is often made with high-fructose corn syrup (likely GMO corn), often with some steps in processing including sulfuric acid or acetone. Gross! Use vitamin C made from food sources like acerola and camu camu (lowest oxalate form of food-based vitamin C). A cherry-size camu camu fruit can contain as much vitamin C as 30 to 60 oranges!
- Supplement with cod liver oil, 1 teaspoon per day, with a meal. This provides retinol, which is a cofactor for ceruloplasmin production. And it's got a ton of other health benefits too.
- Donate blood! Unless you have been diagnosed with hemochromatosis, you will likely not find a practitioner who will give you therapeutic phlebotomy. Many of my clients notice they feel better physically and mentally after donating. Again, a comprehensive blood test is recommended before donating, especially if you are a menstruating woman. For my female clients, I usually recommend doing a blood draw shortly before their period.

- Supplement with magnesium. My favorite forms are magnesium threonate and magnesium sulfate (via Epsom salt soaks).
- Avoid cooking in cast-iron skillets and copper cookware. This is the type of iron and copper that feed the Fenton reaction.
- Eat organic as much as possible. I hit this point in many parts of this book, so I'll just leave it here that crops are often sprayed with a copper-based fungicide.

8.1.1 IRON DYSREGULATION AND ITS EFFECTS ON FERTILITY

It's through the Fenton reaction (discussed throughout Appendix 8) that the hydroxyl radical (•OH) causes oxidative damage to tissues, including the peritoneum, oviduct, and ovary and the follicle, oocyte, sperm, and embryo, potentially impeding embryo development (Máté et al. 2018). Some of the most heartbreaking effects of reactive oxygen species may be the damage to gametes and embryos by damaging the components of the cells that are responsible for coding information and cellular repair. Hydroxyl radicals damage DNA by causing mutations, DNA breaks and fragmentation, and replication impediments and they impair the cell's ability to repair the damage. This damage disrupts the integrity of the genetic code and inheritance for the mitochondrial and nuclear genomes.

NOTE

1 A nerd note for my Nerdies: Since I just mentioned ATP, I want to reiterate that ATP is needed to make SAMe, the universal methyl donor. If our mitochondria are having a hard time making ATP, our SAMe levels will be subpar, and our methylation ability will be low. So, again, we can't blame all methylation issues on MTHFR.

REFERENCES

Dunaief, David, Alyssa Cwanger, and Joshua L. Dunaief. 2014. "Iron-induced retinal damage." *Handbook of Nutrition, Diet and the Eye* 619–626.

Fraser, Stuart T., Robyn G. Midwinter, Birgit S. Berger, and Roland Stocker. 2011. "Heme oxygenase-1: a critical link between iron metabolism, erythropoiesis, and development." *Advances in Hematology*.

Jiang, Rulan, Veronica Lopez, Shannon L. Kelleher, and Bo Lönnerdal. 2011. "Apo-and holo-lactoferrin are both internalized by lactoferrin receptor via clathrin-mediated endocytosis but differentially affect ERK-signaling and cell proliferation in Caco-2 cells." *Journal of Cellular Physiology* 226, no. 11, 3022–3031.

Koricho, Z., G. E. Atomssa, T. C. Mekonnen, and S. E. Tadesse. 2020. "Dietary vitamin A intakes among pregnant women attending antenatal care in health facilities in Dessie Town, North East Ethiopia." *Journal of Human Nutrition and Dietetics* 33, no. 5, 678–685.

Lal, Ashutosh, Wafa Atamna, David W. Killilea, Jung H. Suh, and Bruce N. Ames. 2008. "Lipoic acid and acetyl-carnitine reverse iron-induced oxidative stress in human fibroblasts." *Redox Report* 13, no. 1, 2–10.

Mancinelli, Romina, Luigi Rosa, Antimo Cutone, Maria Stefania Lepanto, Antonio Franchitto, Paolo Onori, Eugenio Gaudio, and Piera Valenti. 2020. "Viral hepatitis and iron dysregulation: molecular pathways and the role of lactoferrin." *Molecules* 25, no. 8, 1997.

Máté, Gábor, Lori R. Bernstein, and Attila L. Török. 2018. "Endometriosis is a cause of infertility: Does reactive oxygen damage to gametes and embryos play a key role in the pathogenesis of infertility caused by endometriosis?" *Frontiers in Endocrinology* 9, 725.

Moayeri, Ardeshir, Ayoob Rostamzadeh, Amir Raoofi, Mohammad Jafar Rezaie, Zahra Abasian, and Reza Ahmadi. 2020. "Retinoic acid and fibroblast growth factor-2 play a key role on modulation of sex hormones and apoptosis in a mouse model of polycystic ovary syndrome induced by estradiol valerate." *Taiwanese Journal of Obstetrics and Gynecology* 59, no. 6, 882–890.

O'Sullivan, Eoin P., and C. Howel Walsh. 2007. "Endocrinopathy of HFE-related hemochromatosis." *Expert Review of Endocrinology & Metabolism* 2, no. 2, 277–286.

Puntarulo, Susana. 2005. "Iron, oxidative stress and human health." *Molecular Aspects of Medicine* 26, no. 4–5, 299–312.

Simcox, Judith A., and Donald A. McClain. 2013. "Iron and diabetes risk." *Cell Metabolism* 17, no. 3, 329–341.

Zhang, Yan, Hailing Li, Yuling Zhao, and Zhonghong Gao. 2006. "Dietary supplementation of baicalin and quercetin attenuates iron overload induced mouse liver injury." *European Journal of Pharmacology* 535, no. 1–3, 236–269.

9 Investigate If Oxalates Are a Culprit

Most things in nature have protective mechanisms to keep from being eaten. Many plants contain compounds that exhibit certain properties that animals inherently know should not be eaten in large quantities. Some of these compounds can rob the body of minerals or much worse. Our ancestors were aware of some of these properties and learned to soak, sprout, ferment, or cook various foods to make them more "digestible." They also ate with the seasons.

It seems only certain cultures and social circles still eat in this manner. Modern humans seem to have lost that innate sense of what is nourishing to the body and what is a burden to the body. And with certain foods readily available 365 days a year, this can actually be a detriment to our health.

Take spinach, for instance. While spinach is a nutrient-dense food, it has an extremely high oxalate (technically, oxalic acid) content and also is a high histamine–containing food. I discuss histamine in Chapter 15. Since learning about oxalates, I firmly believe that our ability to put a handful of spinach in our smoothie every morning could be harming some of us. When our bodies can't effectively deal with oxalates as quickly as they are coming in, they will start to sequester them in various parts of the body.

Oxalates can be produced from yeast and mold. Oxalic acid from foods and/or mold (especially *Aspergillus* and *Penicillium*) interferes with the absorption of minerals by binding to them and forming jagged crystals that can become very painful when they are sequestered in the body. The sharp crystals irritate and shred the surrounding tissues. This is similar to when you get a shard of glass stuck in your foot, and inflammation, fluid, and scar tissue are created to protect the body.

If someone has chronic pain that is not a structural issue, then oxalates should be considered.

Most people have only heard of oxalate crystals in the form of calcium oxalate kidney stones, but they are also associated with interstitial cystitis, vulvodynia, endometriosis, burning urination and/or bowel movements, frequent urination, and recurrent urinary tract infections (UTIs). Pain with intercourse can occur due to the aggregation of oxalates in vaginal tissue.

And if that weren't bad enough, oxalates can get sequestered in many other areas of the body besides the lower abdomen/pelvic bowl. These jagged oxalate crystals can form in places like the joints, muscles, connective tissue (fibromyalgia, anyone?), blood vessels, bones, and brain, causing pain and wreaking havoc on function.

They can be over-absorbed in lung tissue, causing things like pulmonary fibrosis. They can cause vertigo when the crystals get sequestered in the ear canals. (The Epley maneuver can be performed to displace them for symptomatic relief.) They have been found in cataracts in the eyes.

DOI: 10.1201/b23201-11

There are some studies that link oxalates to breast cancer, one even starkly titled "Oxalate Induces Breast Cancer" (Castellaro et al. 2015), so please know that oxalates can lead to very serious consequences if left unaddressed.

A largely unknown fact is that oxalate crystals can get sequestered in the thyroid tissue, causing thyroid issues. One study of autopsies found that 79% of adults had oxalate crystals in their thyroids, with prevalence increasing with age (Reid et al. 1987). To make matters worse, because of the inflammation that oxalates can produce, conversion from T4 to T3 can be hindered, further exacerbating a hypothyroid issue.

Women who experience miscarriage often have thyroid issues. While thyroid disease can be caused by problems with the adrenals or HPA axis, Hashimoto's, or oxalates, thyroid disease is the effect of something and not the *cause* of anything, other than symptoms. We can think of the thyroid as the canary in the coal mine.

A quick note on thyroid testing: Many women are told by their doctors that their thyroids are "fine" when, in fact, they are not functioning optimally. I don't often blog, but I felt compelled to blog about this topic on my website because this is such a common occurrence. The normal range for thyroid markers is much wider than the range for optimal functioning. This causes many women to fall "within normal limits," where "normal limits" are derived from a wide range of blood tests of people who went to the doctor for one reason or another who could very well have had a sluggish thyroid. I'm not going to get into the thyroid-fertility connection here, as there are already lots of great books and articles about this because it is a commonly known factor in impaired fertility. Just know that you want to be certain to get a complete thyroid panel, including thyroid antibodies, and reference them within an optimal functioning range. You can read what these are in a blog on my website, JaclynDowns.com. Also, insulin resistance and chronic blood sugar challenges can overburden thyroid demands, resulting initially in hyperthyroid responses that ultimately exhaust the thyroid and result in hypothyroidism.

Oxalates chelate minerals, depleting them and leading to comorbidities due to loss of minerals that are essential cofactors for enzymatic processes and pH regulation, among many other functions. Because oxalates bind to minerals, osteopenia and osteoporosis can occur since oxalates are stealing the body's calcium. The minerals that are the primary targets of oxalate crystal formation are calcium, magnesium, and iron (which may be beneficial for some folks who have issues with excess iron). Oxalates can also bind to heavy metals, but unlike other chelating agents, oxalates trap heavy metals in the tissues (William Shaw 2015).

Nano-size crystals can get into the cells, causing damage to many parts of the cell, including the membrane and the mitochondria, and can even cause cell necrosis (i.e., cell death). Refer to Chapter 11 on boosting mitochondrial and egg/sperm health.

Poor sulfur tolerance is another symptom of oxalate sensitivity, on which I'll elaborate a little later. But relating to oxalates, many people blame a sensitivity to sulfur foods and substances (i.e., Epsom salt baths, wine, etc.) on a CBS genetic variant, but it could very likely be due to an oxalate sensitivity. This is because oxalates and sulfates have an inverse relationship, sharing and competing for transporters and receptors on the cell (Robijn et al. 2011). When someone boosts their sulfur with an Epsom salt bath, for instance, it can cause oxalate dumping because the sulfate is pushing the oxalates out of the cells and tissues and into the blood, which can make you feel lousy. If you feel worse after doing an Epsom salt bath or foot soak, you may be pushing/mobilizing oxalates out of the cells and tissues faster than your kidneys can filter and excrete them.

An intolerance to sulfur could be a SUOX conversion issue (or other sulfur-related genes – refer to the section on sulfation in Chapter 13 and its related appendix), but for lots of people, it's because the body is overwhelmed with oxalates. SUOX is the gene that turns sulfites into sulfate, which people with variants in this gene may have a reduced capacity to do. Molybdenum, a scarce trace mineral, is a cofactor. Deficiencies in molybdenum will restrict the conversion of sulfites into sulfate and cause other problems.

If you get headaches with sulfur foods or Epsom salt baths, it's not that you don't want to do those wonderful things. It's that you want to go more slowly and add in minerals, especially oral calcium and magnesium, during meals to help bind the oxalic acid in the stomach so you can excrete them in urine and stool. Just like with a low oxalate diet, you can do too much too quickly if you add in too much sulfur too soon.

9.1 A NOTE ON OXALATES AND ESTROGEN DOMINANCE

Oxalates compete with sulfates, which are needed to metabolize hormones. If the body is overrun with oxalates or if you have genetic weaknesses in sulfur-related genes, it will lessen the amount of sulfur the body has for sulfation, which inactivates and detoxifies estrogens, leading to estrogen dominance and paving a smooth road for endometriosis, fibroids, estrogenic cancers, and even thyroid issues, since excess estrogen affects thyroid hormone receptors.

Refer to Appendix 9A for more in-depth information on oxalates and sulfate and DHEA, DHEA-S, aromatase, and urine organic acid test markers related to oxalates.

Some of the highest oxalate foods are some of the most nutritious. The ones that top the list are spinach and beets and their greens, Swiss chard, and rhubarb. Since not many folks regularly eat rhubarb, I usually include sesame seeds on this list – that includes tahini, so that's a heads-up for all you hummus lovers!

As a nutritionist, I never thought that I'd be telling people to stay away from (certain) greens. But yes, there is no one food that is nourishing to every*body*. Bio-individuality is an essential consideration for every client I work with.

The more clients I work with who come to me for impaired fertility and reproductive health, the more I see oxalate issues, but this is not saying that they are a concern for everyone and that you should avoid eating these extremely nutritious foods!

There are conditions called "primary hyperoxaluria" and "secondary hyperoxaluria." The primary form involves genetic polymorphisms of the HOGA1, AGXT, SPP1, and/or GRHPR genes, creating defective enzyme activity, which prevents normal metabolism of oxalates. Refer to Appendix 9B for more information on these genes.

Secondary hyperoxaluria can be from things like overuse of antibiotics or prolonged mold exposure (see Chapter 7), which can easily become systemic. Secondary hyperoxaluria also goes hand in hand with issues with fat utilization, which, in an upcoming chapter, I will expand on how fat utilization issues can cause impaired fertility.

Oxalates can be obtained from three sources: liver cells (our bodies produce oxalates endogenously in the last turn of the Krebs cycle), yeast species, and food.

Compromised gut health plays a large part in oxalate sensitivity and poor oxalate metabolism. If someone has intestinal permeability, otherwise known as "leaky gut," the oxalates are able to easily pass through the tight junctions that secure the intestinal wall and enter the bloodstream.

I already mentioned candida overgrowth (an opportunistic anaerobe) being one cause of oxalates. When someone has dysbiosis (an imbalance between good and bad gut bacteria, with fungal growth typically thrown into the mix), they do not have enough good bacteria to help with oxalate degradation.

There is a form of bacteria known to degrade oxalates, and it is *Oxalobacter formigenes*. Unfortunately, the supplement form is not yet available for sale in the United States.

Poor fat digestion (see Chapter 10) and absorption are also contributing factors. In fact, the number one documented cause of hyperoxaluria is poor fat digestion. We need to bind oxalic acid with calcium in the digestive tract to excrete it harmlessly in stool. If we are not emulsifying and using fats, they will instead get bound up with the calcium and get excreted, leaving the oxalates to run amok.

So if you have gallbladder dysfunction, bile flow issues, or emulsification issues, you can have over-absorption of oxalates. You may have issues with oxalate absorption if you have any of the below symptoms of fat utilization issues:

- Discomfort from and/or poor digestion of fatty foods
- Oily stools (seeing oil on top of the toilet water, just like seeing it on a puddle in a parking lot on a rainy day)
- "Skid marks" left after flushing
- Pale, clay-colored stools
- Floating stools
- Fecal fat in a stool test
- Elevated markers for fat utilization on a urine organic acids test

Addressing fat maldigestion and utilization issues is a first step when dealing with oxalate issues.

Oxalates can make you feel crappy emotionally as well. They are associated with depression for a few reasons. First, if they mess up your gut health and your gut-brain interconnectivity, your nutrient absorption will be subpar, and you won't have the nutrients (or beneficial bacteria) to act as cofactors for neurotransmitter production and metabolism.

Also, you have more neurotransmitter receptors in your gut than in your brain. Combine that with the fact that a majority of your neurotransmitters are produced and housed in the gut, so that balance will be off. Plus, neurotransmitters are proteins, which are made of amino acids. If you are not properly digesting your proteins (the most difficult macromolecule breakdown), they won't get broken down into amino acids, and other proteins cannot be assembled (i.e., impaired protein metabolism). And inflammation is characterized by "undigested proteins," which is why proteolytic/systemic enzymes help lower inflammation. Plus, inflammation and depression are closely related (Giovanni et al. 2017), and issues with oxalates are a major source of inflammation. And finally, oxalates chelate magnesium, which is needed for optimal neurological functioning.

ACTION STEPS

What can you do if you suspect or confirm with testing that oxalates are an issue for you?

- Ensure that it is not a mold/mycotoxin issue that is causing or exacerbating your oxalate sensitivity. Refer to Chapter 7 on mold/mycotoxins.
- Check your vitamin B6 status via a urine organic acid test, as B6 is the primary metabolite for the conversion of glycolic acid to glycine. When there is a deficiency of B6, glycolic acid is instead converted to oxalate. I highly recommend supplementing with the P5P form, as it is a bioavailable form of B6. Also, regarding testing, I prefer urine to blood testing when investigating B vitamin status. Here is an example of why: Many people go to the doctor because they experience fatigue. The doctor draws blood and checks the B12 levels, which look fine. Oftentimes, B12 gets stuck in the blood because there are issues with transport or absorption (which can be due to SNPs in TCN or GIF genes, among others). If B12 isn't able to get into the cells to be utilized and properly metabolized, then of course the blood levels are going to look ample, especially in meat eaters. Urine is like a car's exhaust; it tells us what the body has utilized and is now getting rid of. Regarding hormones and B6, B6 helps regulate hormone activity, increasing progesterone and throwing the hammer down on estrogen dominance.
- Supplement with minerals, especially calcium and magnesium, *with meals.* Always take those minerals with food so they can bind to oxalates in the digestive tract and be excreted in stool. Otherwise, if calcium is taken without food, it gets into the bloodstream where it can bind with oxalates, causing calcium oxalate crystals to form in various parts of the body. You can use calcium citrate, potassium citrate, or magnesium orotate to increase oxalate excretion. Note: If you do supplement with calcium outside mealtime (which I rarely recommend), I encourage you to take it with vitamin K2. K2 helps usher the calcium into the bones where it belongs, rather than it getting deposited in the arteries and creating plaque.

The minerals will act as binders for the oxalates, binding them in the gut to be excreted so they are not able to bind with oxalates in the blood and wreak their havoc. I specify the citrate form of potassium and/or calcium because studies have identified low citrate levels as a cause of secondary hyperoxaluria, and citrate is a well-known inhibitor of calcium oxalate crystallization (Byer and Khan 2005). You can use magnesium citrate as well, but some people speculate that magnesium citrate may inhibit ceruloplasmin production, which I detailed in Chapter 8.

- Take Epsom salt baths. Epsom salts are simply magnesium sulfate. You get the benefits of both magnesium and sulfate. Remember that sulfate will crowd out the oxalates in the cell. If you are not into baths, feel free to do foot soaks. A little bit ago I mentioned Epsom salt baths and how they can cause reactions with oxalates. Just like with the diet, we can do too much too quickly and cause dumping, so start slow and low and titrate up as tolerated by your body. You should feel nothing but relaxed afterwards.
- Supplement with MSM (methylsulfonylmethane) either in pill form or topically. It is rich in sulfate.
- Fix your gut! While the recommendations in this chapter can help with management, fixing the gut is getting at the root system. Remember, aside from the intake of air and water, digestion is the most important step in metabolism; it turns "not you" (i.e., food) into "you." Therefore, addressing and promoting optimal gut health will improve overall health and help lower oxalates. This means getting rid of yeast/fungus, improving fat utilization, and sealing the leaky tight junctions.
- Eliminate the highest food sources of oxalates and follow a low-oxalate diet. I cannot emphasize enough that this should be done g-r-a-d-u-a-l-l-y to prevent oxalate "dumping," which is when the oxalates get rapidly released out of sequestration mode and into the blood. The rule of thumb is to reduce by 5–10% each week. Personally, I recommend just eliminating the top foods I mentioned and start with only taking minerals with each meal, depending on how crazy your oxalate load may be. The goal for chronic stone formers is 50mg per day total, which is insanely low, although it takes a long time to reach that low of a level, and most people don't need to be that restrictive.

Appendix 9C briefly discusses the relationship between mast cell activation and urine organic acid test markers that can indicate oxalate issues.

When I discussed iron dysregulation and true anemia, I stated that they usually only occur if someone has a bleeding disorder or is vegan. Well, when excessive amounts of oxalates bind to iron, this can also be a cause of anemia.

I want to repeat that I don't want to scare people away from eating foods that are high in oxalates because many of them are extremely healthy. I just wanted to let you know, dear reader, about how oxalates can wreak havoc on the body, and what clues to look for to know if this is happening. Consider it a very large rock that should be looked under in anyone's fertility journey.

REFERENCES

Byer, Karen, and Saeed R. Khan. 2005. "Citrate provides protection against oxalate and calcium oxalate crystal induced oxidative damage to renal epithelium." *The Journal of Urology* 173, no. 2, 640–646.

Castellaro, Andrés M., Alfredo Tonda, Hugo H. Cejas, Héctor Ferreyra, Beatriz L. Caputto, Oscar A. Pucci, and German A. Gil. 2015. "Oxalate induces breast cancer." *BMC Cancer* 15, no. 1, 1–13.

Giovanni, Amodeo, Maria Allegra Trusso, and Andrea Fagiolini. 2017. "Depression and inflammation: Disentangling a clear yet complex and multifaceted link." *Neuropsychiatry* 7, no. 4, 448–457.

Reid, John D., Chang-Hyun Choi, and Norman O. Oldroyd. 1987. "Calcium oxalate crystals in the thyroid: Their identification, prevalence, origin, and possible significance." *American Journal of Clinical Pathology* 87, no. 4, 443–454.

Robijn, Stef, Bernd Hoppe, Benjamin A. Vervaet, Patrick C. D'haese, and Anja Verhulst. 2011. "Hyperoxaluria: A gut-kidney axis?" *Kidney International* 80, no. 11, 1146–1158.

William, Shaw. 2015. *Great Plains Laboratory*, November 16. www.greatplainslaboratory.com/articles-1/2015/11/13/oxalates-control-is-a-major-new-factor-in-autism-therapy.

10 The Importance of Proper Fat Utilization for Hormonal Balance and Fetal Growth

Cholesterol has been vilified for decades now, and people think it's good to get their cholesterol as low as possible. What many people don't realize is that cholesterol is the precursor to steroid hormones in the body. This means our sex/reproductive hormones, our stress hormones, and even vitamin D are completely dependent upon cholesterol. Cholesterol also plays a major role in creating healthy bile.

Without going off on too much of a tangent, I will state that elevated cholesterol is often due to too many sugars and refined carbs. Elevated cholesterol is also a panic-stricken defense response to a deficiency in vitamin D, which is made from cholesterol. I also know it can be caused by sulfate insufficiency since cholesterol that is sulfated is water soluble and is therefore able to travel freely in the blood, rather than being packaged up inside an LDL particle. I discuss sulfation in the chapters on oxalates and phase 2 liver detoxification. Stephanie Seneff, triple PhD and senior research scientist at MIT, discusses sulfate in great detail and refers to it as "the most common nutritional deficiency you have never heard of."

Fats are necessary to synthesize hormones and clear old hormones from the body. Healthy fats and the proper digestion/utilization of them play enormous roles in maintaining health that extend beyond hormonal balance. Here are just a few things that fats are needed for:

- Brain health (Our brains are 80% fat.)
- Neuroprotection (The Myelin sheath is the fatty coating that protects our neurons.)
- Immune system functioning
- Blood sugar stability
- Healthy skin and hair

Healthy fats serve as a fuel source for our bodies and are essential components of cell membranes. This includes mitochondrial membranes.

If we are not utilizing or absorbing our fats, the fat-soluble vitamins A, D, E, and K will not be able to benefit our bodies! Same with the good fats like butter, avocado, cod liver oil, and omega 3s. If we are not properly digesting, absorbing, or utilizing our fats, they can create problems with all the things they are used for (listed earlier), and they can create especially bad free radicals through a process called lipid peroxidation.

DOI: 10.1201/b23201-12

Our gallbladders are essential for proper fat utilization. They store the bile that the liver produces and secrete it as needed to emulsify fats into tiny globules in order to absorb all the good fats we need.

Bile is super critical for a healthy, functioning body. Not only is it required for proper fat digestion and utilization, but it also regulates glucose and cholesterol metabolism. Activation of thyroid hormones is dependent on bile flow as well. Bile salts are rich in choline which is one reason they affect the microbiome and enhance gastrointestinal motility (Shade and Decker n.d.).

It is unfortunate that cholecystectomy is one of the most common surgeries in the United States. Fat malabsorption can cause hormonal imbalance and is the primary cause of gallstones and gallbladder pain. The irony is that without gallbladders, the potential for hormonal imbalance is increased dramatically. This is sad because fat malabsorption can be greatly improved through a few simple protocols. If you have had your gallbladder removed, it is recommended to supplement ox bile or TUDCA (a derivative of bile acid) with meals.

Bile flow is key for fat utilization. Hormone health is all about the bile!

Here's how fat digestion works, if everything is working properly:

The liver synthesizes bile and bile acids from cholesterol (another reason cholesterol isn't the bad guy). The liver sends toxins and used hormones into the bile. Then it ships the bile to the gallbladder. The gallbladder stores bile and secretes it into the small intestine when we eat a meal that contains fat. The bile breaks down the fat so we can absorb it, and then the toxins in the bile exit the body with the feces.

Bile flow is tremendously inhibited in states of stress or, more technically, when our autonomic nervous system is in sympathetic dominance ("fight, flight, or freeze" mode). Again, from an evolutionary perspective, when we are running from a bear, we aren't stopping to eat. We are using all our bodily energies to get us away from the stressor, so we definitely do not want to waste energy on digesting. In relation to the "freeze" mode, instead of running, sometimes all our bodies can do is shut down, or "freeze" in order to be able to deal with a stressor. Either way, bile doesn't flow well in this sympathetic state.

Supporting healthy bile production and secretion is essential for healthy fat utilization. If bile is thick and sludgy, it will not flow easily and won't be able to properly break down fats, causing our brain health and hormone production to pay the price. If bile isn't flowing, then toxins (almost all of which are lipophilic [attracted to fats]) and "dirty" hormones aren't being cleared from the body either.

And if there are also issues with fat digestion, then the problem is compounded.

Symptoms of fat malabsorption:

- Floating stools
- Light-colored stools
- "Oil slicks" on top of toilet water with bowel movement
- "Skid marks" after flushing
- Dry skin (I tell my clients that water is hydration for the body; fats are lubrication.)
- Gallbladder pain (under lower ribs on right side) or gallstones
- Nausea after eating
- Hormone imbalance and the symptoms that accompany it

The Great Plains urine organic acids test measures seven markers for fatty acid oxidation and can tell us if fats are not properly utilized and to what degree.

10.1 THE FAT/OXALATE RELATIONSHIP

I want to reiterate what I stated in the chapter on oxalates: When there are gallbladder or fat utilization issues, the improperly used fats will bind to minerals, like calcium, in the gut (limiting calcium from binding to oxalates) and will be eliminated in the stool, leaving oxalates to run amok. So, potentially, issues with oxalates can be symptomatic of fat utilization issues.

10.2 L-CARNITINE TO THE RESCUE!

L-Carnitine is an amino acid that plays an important role in fatty acid metabolism and energy production.

L-Carnitine is essential for fertility because it is needed for so many functions.

A fantastic article in *Reproductive Biology and Endocrinology*, titled "Role of L-Carnitine in Female Infertility" shares a ton of info on how L-carnitine and the acetylated form, acetyl-L-carnitine, play important roles in fertility and reproductive issues (Agarwal et al. 2018). The article discusses how oxidative stress negatively affects lipid peroxidation of oocytes, as well as fertilization and embryo development in animals.

It also discusses how carnitine has been used to enhance ART treatments and can improve oocyte health and overall sperm health by ameliorating the effects of oxidative stress and enhancing cellular membrane stability and energy production "to maintain the robustness of reproductive cells."

It states that studies have indicated that decreased levels of L-carnitine are strongly correlated to alterations in insulin and sex hormones and that supplementation with both forms can improve PCOS and amenorrhea and may improve endometriosis.

NADPH (discussed extensively in Chapter 11) is needed for protection from oxidative stress in a high-fat diet. Someone doing a high-fat or keto diet with low NADPH will likely experience an increase in inflammation and oxidative stress and increase in LDL cholesterol and will, therefore, feel markedly worse, not better/clearer. Also, one should have good carnitine transport and choline status to ensure proper usage of fats before doing a high-fat/ketogenic diet. There can be genetic variants in genes like SLC22A5, PEMT, and ACAT that hinder proper fat transport and metabolism.

Clinical pearl: Because the glucuronidation pathway (a phase 2 liver detoxification pathway that clears a ton of substances) requires glucose, if someone has any genetic variants in the genes related to glucuronidation (notably the UGT genes), they may want to consider pulsing ketogenic diets, as opposed to doing them long term. Refer to Chapter 13 to learn more about the glucuronidation pathway.

What's the basic difference between acetyl-L-Carnitine and L-Carnitine?

When deciding which form of carnitine to supplement, you will, of course, ask this question. The biggest differences between the two are that L-carnitine is most commonly used for fat burning and energy production by turning triglycerides into fuel. On the other hand, acetyl-L-carnitine is most often associated with anti-aging and antioxidant effects, can cross the blood-brain-barrier, and is more readily absorbed by the gut. Plus, the acetylated form has the acetyl group that can be beneficial for the phase 2 liver detoxification pathway of acetylation (which I discuss in Chapter 13).

10.3 OTHER HELPFUL NUTRIENTS FOR PROPER FAT USAGE

Choline!

When it comes to getting or being pregnant, folate gets the spotlight, but choline needs to get some time on the mic.

One of choline's primary jobs is to support lipid transport. It also plays a huge part in neurotransmitter synthesis, cell structure, and cell membranes, along with their signaling. Deficiency has been associated with non-alcoholic fatty liver disease (NAFLD) and atherosclerosis.

Choline circulates the central nervous system, and it plays important roles in brain and memory development in the fetus. Studies show it appears to decrease the risk of the development of neural tube defects (Shaw et al. 2004; Imbard et al. 2013).

Several studies have demonstrated that adequate choline supplementation can prevent preterm birth, preeclampsia, fetal loss, and/or growth restriction by regulating inflammation (Zhang et al. 2018). My absolute favorite form is phosphatidylcholine (PC), especially in liposomal form. (Quicksilver Scientific is the brand I use and recommend.) Inflammation during pregnancy is known to produce many adverse reactions and outcomes, including spontaneous abortion, preterm birth, intrauterine growth restriction (IUGR), and preeclampsia (Zhang et al. 2018). But you already knew from reading this book that inflammation causes reproductive difficulties, right?

The need for choline increases considerably during pregnancy, as it is critical to fetal and placental growth and has a modulatory role in the fetal epigenome. It influences stem cell proliferation and apoptosis, thereby altering brain and spinal cord structure and function and influencing risk for neural tube defects and lifelong memory function (Zeisel 2006).

A review in *Trends in Endocrinology & Metabolism* states that maternal choline supplementation during pregnancy benefits important physiologic systems such as offspring cognitive function, response to stress, and cerebral inhibition and that it may improve the lifelong health of the child (Jiang et al. 2014).

Choline is a "conditionally essential nutrient," which means that it serves an indispensable physiologic function and that our bodies can make certain amounts, but it may also require supplementation through diet and supplements. Increased requirements can be due to absorption issues, pregnancy, lactation, and common genetic polymorphisms (Zeisel and Da Costa 2009).

It is only the PEMT gene that makes the enzyme that synthesizes choline. More specifically, the enzyme phosphatidylethanolamine *N*-methyltransferase (PEMT) makes phosphatidylcholine in the liver. Genetic polymorphisms in the PEMT gene will slow down its production, which can increase the predisposition for fatty liver disease.

The important point to emphasize here is that the PEMT gene is fueled by estrogen, so women of reproductive age tend to make more choline. This biological mastery makes sense since estrogen levels are up to 30 times higher in pregnancy, allowing for more choline to be produced, which is critical to fetal development and a successful pregnancy.

PEMT variants can create an ineffective response to estrogen. Even if a woman of reproductive age has high estrogen levels, if she has PEMT variants, she may still be susceptible to choline deficiency, especially if she is not getting an adequate amount through dietary sources or supplementation.

In this book, I detail how important insulin sensitivity, liver detox ability, and fatty acid metabolism are for hormonal balance. Choline assists with all these things! This is one reason choline is often recommended for PCOS and fertility support: because it helps manage insulin levels and assist fat metabolism.

Refer to the Appendix 10 visual and caption for information on choline and the major part it plays in the methylation pathway.

Choline helps keep the liver and gallbladder healthy. It is a primary component of bile, which is needed to absorb fat-soluble vitamins. It is important for conjugating toxins to excrete in the stool. If we don't have enough choline, our liver and gallbladder activity can become stagnant. On a side note, I have often wondered how many people with PEMT variants have had their gallbladders removed when some extra choline might have helped prevent the issues leading up to removal.

I mentioned earlier that choline is critical for cell membrane integrity (it is involved in constructing the phospholipid bilayer [cell membrane] of all the cells in all the soft tissues of the body), and you're making a lot of cells when you're growing a baby! Don't wait until you get a big fat positive pregnancy test. The rapidly dividing organism that is your growing child needs all these nutrients far before a pregnancy test can notify you of good news.

The benefits of choline don't stop once you give birth; choline is concentrated in breast milk as it is crucial for a baby's developing cells, brain, and organs.

According to an article in the *Journal of the American College of Nutrition* titled "Nutritional Importance of Choline for Brain Development," the foods highest in total choline concentrations per 100g were beef liver (418 mg), chicken liver (290 mg), and eggs (251 mg) (Zeisel 2004).

ACTION STEPS

Making sure fats are properly digested and utilized is essential for healthy fertility and fetal growth. Anything that supports bile flow will be helpful in fat utilization. These are my top picks for improving fat digestion and utilization, and for supporting bile flow:

- Phosphatidylcholine helps prevent 'sludgy' bile and the formation of gallstones. Some rich food sources are egg yolks, sunflower lecithin, and wild-caught fish.
- Ox bile can be a great supplement, but we want to empower your body to make it, not depend on a supplement. This is why I don't recommend it long term unless you've had your gallbladder removed.
- TUDCA (tauroursodeoxycholic acid) is a water-soluble component of bile acid that allows for better digestion of fats. Again, maybe not a long-term solution unless you've had your gallbladder removed.

- Bitters are a great herbal way to support digestion and stimulate bile flow, the liver, and the gallbladder. A few common bitter herbs are dandelion root, artichoke leaf, gentian, hops, and barberry. I love Quicksilver Scientific's BitterX.
- For fat digestion, lipase is a digestive enzyme that breaks down lipids. Keep in mind that lipase works on emulsified fats, so bile production and flow should be addressed before lipase is used.
- Improve overall digestion with hydrochloric acid. This will ensure the stomach is able to signal for the pancreas to make pancreatic enzymes that help with fat utilization and absorption.
- Riboflavin (vitamin B2) helps break down fats, as well as protein and carbohydrates, so they can be used for fuel. Studies have found that riboflavin deficiency is associated with an increased risk of preeclampsia in pregnant women. I want to note that riboflavin is also needed for folate and pyridoxine (vitamin B6) to be activated. It is a cofactor for the MTHFR enzyme. I prefer the R-5-P form.
- Castor oil packs not only support liver/gallbladder health but also support healthy hormonal balance, digestion and gut health, movement of lymph, and detoxification. These packs are placed over the liver/gallbladder area of the abdomen, around the bottom of the right-side ribs. A hot water bottle is then applied, and the oil is absorbed into lymphatic circulation, providing a relaxing, cleansing, and anti-inflammatory treatment. Castor oil packs also work wonders for fertility and menstrual issues when placed over the lower abdomen. These have been shown to be helpful for fibroids, PCOS, endometriosis, and all things PMS related. Do not use these if there is a chance of pregnancy. Refer to the resources section for my top recommendation for castor oil, packs, and kits.

REFERENCES

Agarwal, Ashok, Pallav Sengupta, and Damayanthi Durairajanayagam. 2018. "Role of L-carnitine in female infertility." *Reproductive Biology and Endocrinology* 16, no. 1, 1–18.

Imbard, Apolline, Jean-François Benoist, and Henk J. Blom. 2013. "Neural tube defects, folic acid and methylation." *International Journal of Environmental Research and Public Health* 10, no. 9, 4352–4389.

Jiang, Xinyin, Allyson A. West, and Marie A. Caudill. 2014. "Maternal choline supplementation: a nutritional approach for improving offspring health?" *Trends in Endocrinology & Metabolism* 25, no. 5, 263–273.

Shade, Christopher, and Carrie Decker. n.d. *Townsend Letter.* www.townsendletter.com/article/a-push-catch-system-that-enables-effective-detoxification/.

Shaw, Gary M., Suzan L. Carmichael, Wei Yang, Steve Selvin, and Donna M. Schaffer. 2004. "Periconceptional dietary intake of choline and betaine and neural tube defects in offspring." *American Journal of Epidemiology* 160, no. 2, 102–109.

Zeisel, Steven H. 2004. "Nutritional importance of choline for brain development." *Journal of the American College of Nutrition* 23, no. 6, 621S–626S.

Zeisel, Steven H. 2006. "Choline: critical role during fetal development and dietary requirements in adults." *Annual Review of Nutrition* 26, 229–250.

Zeisel, Steven H., and Kerry-Ann Da Costa. 2009. "Choline: an essential nutrient for public health." *Nutrition Reviews* 67, no. 11, 615–623.

Zhang, Min, Xinjia Han, Juejie Bao, Jinying Yang, Shao-Qing Shi, Robert E. Garfield, and Huishu Liu. 2018. "Choline supplementation during pregnancy protects against gestational lipopolysaccharide-induced inflammatory responses." *Reproductive Sciences* 25, no. 1, 74–85.

11 Improve Egg and Sperm Health

We cannot talk about egg and sperm health without discussing mitochondria, just as we cannot talk about oxidative stress without the discussion of antioxidants. In Chapter 2, I defined oxidative stress and antioxidants. I wrote about glutathione, superoxide dismutase (SOD), and catalase and how they function in the body. In this chapter's related appendix (Appendix 11), I dive much deeper into the genes and substances that govern production, utilization, and recycling of these antioxidants.

This chapter (and the related appendix) discusses the functional pathways of antioxidants and how they are central to a seemingly endless number of processes in the body. This will get biochemical, and you may get bored. If so, skim through the chapter/appendix, see what jumps out at you, and leave the rest. The bottom line is that anything that supports cellular (including egg and sperm) health and longevity will benefit fertility.

Before I get to that, I want to cover the basics on boosting mitochondrial health. Most of the things I discuss in the book help boost mitochondrial health, but directly supporting our mighty mitochondria will enhance the functional benefits of and make the most impact in improving egg and sperm quality.

I wrote in Chapter 1 that the mitochondria are the only source of energy that the egg has, and the quality of the egg is the determining factor in achieving a successful pregnancy.

Mitochondrial DNA (mtDNA) is a type of DNA located in the cytoplasm (as opposed to the nucleus, where DNA resides) and inside the mitochondria. Mitochondrial concentrations vary based on a cell's need for energy. For example, a thumb muscle cell may have 6 to 10 mitochondria per cell; a heart cell can contain 600 to 1,000 mitochondria per cell; and brain cells can contain up to 30,000 mitochondria per cell. In humans, the mature egg cell, or oocyte, contains the highest number of mitochondria among human cells, ranging from 100,000 to 600,000 mitochondria per cell (Haskett 2014). In contrast, human sperm have on average 50 to 75. The number and health of the mitochondria affect embryonic growth and development. All those mitochondria are there in the event that the egg gets fertilized so that the zygote/blastocyst/embryo/fetus has enough energy to carry it throughout the early stages of development (Figure 11.1).

DOI: 10.1201/b23201-13

Mitochondria

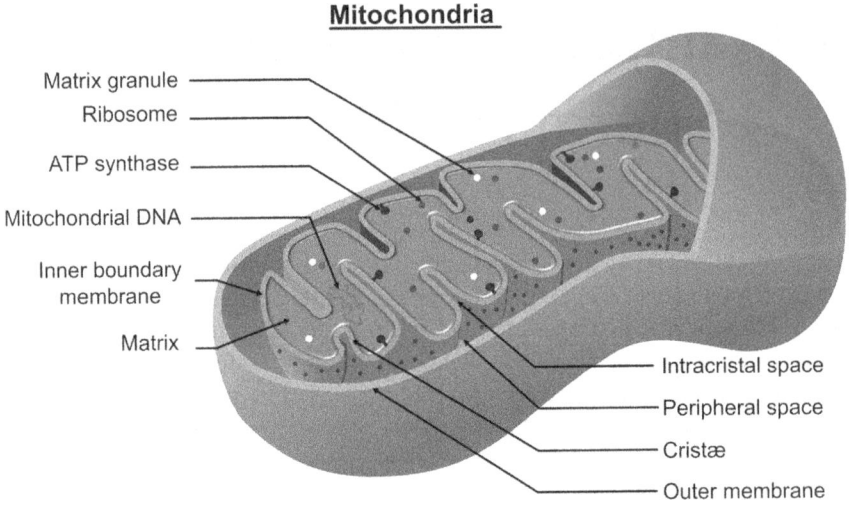

FIGURE 11.1   Diagram and anatomy of mitochondria.

I want to emphasize the importance of the mitochondria, which make ATP (cellular currency for energy production). Mitochondria affect all aspects of mammalian reproduction (Babayev and Seli 2015) and are particularly susceptible to oxidative stress. The maturation and quality of our eggs are heavily reliant on optimally functioning mitochondria, and so are fertilization and embryonic development (Tatone et al. 2015). When we have mitochondrial dysfunction, the eggs and/or sperm will not be of prime quality and will not have enough energy to ensure proper chromosome and cell division. This can result in embryos with chromosomal abnormalities. As far as we currently know, it is only the mother who passes mitochondria – specifically, mitochondrial DNA – to offspring via the egg. I'd like to note that ART procedures affect mitochondrial function, so providing support with mitochondrial nutrients may increase mitochondrial performance in eggs (Babayev and Seli 2015). If the body can't make energy, then it definitely will switch off mating ability because that requires a tremendous amount of energy. Mitochondrial damage can easily happen and affects every cell, tissue, organ, and system in the body.

A professor of genetics in the departments of medicine, pediatrics, and pathology at UCSD, Robert K. Naviaux, describes this response as the cell danger response (CDR). I have called it a survival panic-induced response: that is, a metabolic response that protects cells and hosts from harm and controls innate immunity and healing. Mitochondria regulate the cell danger response that is triggered by encounters with chemical, physical, emotional, or biological threats that exceed the cellular capacity for homeostasis (Naviaux 2020). This basically means that the cell danger response kicks on when there is more stress than the cell can handle and the cell switches from growth and reproduction mode into self-defense mode. When it comes to mitochondrial research and understanding, Robert Naviaux, MD, PhD, is the master, in my opinion.

In his article in the journal *Mitochondrion* titled "Perspective: Cell danger response Biology – The new science that connects environmental health with mitochondria and the rising tide of chronic illness," Naviaux states that chemical pollutants in the environment lower the threshold for CDR activation and:

> Persistent activation of CDR inhibits healing and leads to chronic illness. Once triggered, healing cannot be completed until the choreographed stages of the CDR are returned to an updated state of readiness. Although the CDR is a cellular response, it has the power to change human thought and behavior, child development, physical fitness and resilience, fertility, and the susceptibility of entire populations to disease. Mitochondria regulate the CDR by monitoring and responding to the physical, chemical, and microbial conditions within and around the cell. In this way, mitochondria connect cellular health to environmental health.
>
> (Naviaux 2020)

Mitochondrial functioning decreases as women age, in large part due to the factors that I highlight in this book. "Older eggs" may be able to create just enough ATP to support fertilization and the early stages of embryonic development but may not have quite the capacity to sustain it before implantation takes place (Reader et al. 2017). Supporting optimal functioning of the mitochondria will improve cell health (including egg and sperm), which will lead to improved reproductive capacity and overall health.

Luckily, we can measure some degree of mitochondrial health in a urine organic acids test (OAT). Great Plains Laboratory measures nine markers, which can give your practitioner a good idea of how your mitochondria may be functioning. I especially love this test because it has three markers for oxalate metabolism. I want to declare that I have no affiliation with Great Plains Lab; I just think they are a phenomenal testing company that is up on cutting-edge information. There are other methods for assessing mitochondrial functioning, but this is the test that I use.

In this book, I provide action steps that everyone can implement for their health, all of which will impact the health of mitochondria. Here are some that are known to be beneficial to mitochondria.

ACTION STEPS

Some super-supportive nutrients for mighty mitochondria are:

- B vitamins. B vitamins play an essential role in maintaining mitochondrial function, and mitochondria are compromised by a deficiency in any B vitamin. They also prevent mitochondrial toxicity and act as antioxidants, preventing oxidative stress (Depeint et al. 2006).
- CoQ10. Coenzyme Q10 (also called ubiquinone and ubiquinol) has numerous benefits, especially for mitochondrial function in the egg cells. Studies show that CoQ10 can reverse age-related decline in egg quality (Ben-Meir et al. 2015). It also increases sperm count and motility. CoQ10 is likened to the 'spark plug' of the cell and carries electrons through the electron transport chain to make ATP, so deficiency equals decreased ATP production and also oxidative damage from increased electron loss (Pizzorno 2014). The top food sources of CoQ10 are organ meat (like heart and liver),

oily fish, whole grains, avocados, olives, and broccoli. If you aren't eating CoQ10 rich foods, consider supplementing.

- D-ribose. D-ribose is a non-glycemic simple sugar found in every cell of your body. It is essential for energy production. Supplemental D-ribose has been shown to improve cellular processes when there is mitochondrial dysfunction. Not only is it part of the structure of the ATP molecule, D-ribose is also part of the genetic materials deoxyribonucleic acid (DNA) and ribonucleic acid (RNA).

- Vitamin E is a naturally occurring antioxidant that is shown in animal studies to protect mitochondria from oxidative stress. Vitamin E's actual name is 'tocopherol,' derived from the ancient Greek words τόκος, meaning childbirth, and *pheros*, meaning "to carry, bear, or bring forth." The "-ol" ending signifies its status as a chemical alcohol. Nuts and seeds, especially sunflower seeds, are great food sources of vitamin E.

- NMN and NR. Nicotinamide mononucleotide and nicotinamide riboside are precursors to NAD+. I discuss these forms of vitamin B3 (niacin) in Appendix 11 and go into nerdy detail about them and NAD+. In the 1940s, NR was first shown to raise levels of NAD+ far more efficiently than niacin. As precursors to NAD+, NMN and NR provide a wondrous amount of benefit to the body, boosting this anti-aging molecule, but let's just discuss how they pertain to fertility. NMN supplementation has been shown to "efficaciously improve the quality of oocytes from naturally aged mice by recovering nicotinamide adenine dinucleotide (NAD+) levels" (Miao et al. 2020). NMN also increases ovulation, fertilization, and embryonic development. It does this by restoring mitochondrial function and eliminating reactive oxygen species (ROS)/free radicals. One study's summary puts it succinctly: "Collectively, our data reveal that NMN supplementation is a feasible approach to protect oocytes from advanced maternal age-related deterioration, contributing to the improvement of reproductive outcome of aged women and assisted reproductive technology" (Miao et al. 2020). Studies show that not only can NMN rejuvenate egg quality in older animals, leading to a restoration in fertility, but the benefits also "extend to the developing embryo, where supplementation reverses the adverse effect of maternal age on developmental milestones" (Bertoldo et al. 2020).

- Alpha-lipoic acid (ALA) and acetyl-L-carnitine (ALC). While each on its own has numerous, hugely positive benefits, when taken together, a synergistic effect occurs. When taken together, ALA and ALC increase mitochondrial ATP production (Pizzorno 2014). One paper in the journal *Human Reproduction* showed that when these nutrients were taken in combination with N-acetyl L-cysteine, they cause faster development from the two-cell stage through to the expanded blastocyst stage, accompanied by a significant increase in blastocyst cell numbers and a reduction of intracellular hydrogen peroxide (H_2O_2) levels. (H_2O_2 is discussed in the chapter on iron dysregulation.) The study concludes by saying that supplementation of antioxidants to the IVF medium, as well as to embryo cultures, may further assist in maintaining the viability of human embryos in ART, conceivable through the reduction of oxidative stress (Truong and Gardner 2017).

- PQQ. Mice studies have shown PQQ to protect mitochondria from oxidative stress and stimulate mitochondrial biogenesis (Saihara et al. 2017). This means that it induces the growth of new mitochondria. It also has been shown to activate SIRT1 (the importance of SIRT genes and how they relate to fertility and longevity are discussed in Appendix 11) by increasing cellular levels of NAD+. Although there aren't a whole lot of human studies, research is showing a synergistic effect on fertility with PQQ combined with CoQ10.

LIFESTYLE ACTION STEPS TO SUPPORT MITOCHONDRIA

- Exercise and build muscle mass. Strength training, even among those with mitochondrial damage, has been shown to increase ATP production and mitochondrial function.
- Decrease toxin exposure. At the beginning of this chapter, I discussed how toxins affect the cell danger response and mitochondrial energy production. I also have written a chapter about how toxins impact our bodies (Chapter 12). One game-like way to start decreasing toxic exposures is through the DetoxMe app. There are also plenty of books and blogs that offer tips, tricks, and hacks to get you living a more toxin-free lifestyle.
- Avoid drugs that damage mitochondria. While there are a bunch of prescription medications that are known to damage mitochondria, I'm not telling you to get off those! That's for you to discuss with your doctor. However, there are some over-the-counter (OTC) drugs that can negatively affect your mitochondria: namely acetaminophen, aspirin, and NSAIDS. Go through your medicine cabinet and get rid of any that you can. Chances are there's a natural alternative. While antibiotics are known to damage mitochondria, I'm not saying never to take them. In each case, weigh the risk/benefit of antibiotics before taking them.
- Photobiomodulation, also known as "red light therapy" and low-level laser light therapy (LLLT), has been shown to boost mitochondrial function and ATP production; lower inflammation, which protects the eggs and sperm from oxidative stress; and improve circulation throughout the pelvic area. It also has been shown to decrease stress/promote parasympathetic nervous system function, speed tissue healing, and soften scarring and adhesions. You can find these devices in clinics and for sale online for home use, but their capacities for effectiveness vary widely. In my home, I use Platinum LED Bio, which my electrical engineer husband chose for me when I asked for one for my birthday. Refer to the Resources page for more information about this product and other red light therapy options. There are also tutorials online on how to make your own device for much less money. The home systems like this are more for lowering inflammation and overall health and won't be very effective as a direct follicle booster

because they will not be able to reach the follicles to impact the egg's mitochondria.

I asked Dr. Lorne Brown, clinical director of Acubalance Wellness Centre in Vancouver, British Columbia, and pioneer of the Laser Baby Program (and author of this book's Foreword), the difference between the photobiomodulation systems in some clinics like his and the home systems available on the markets (like mine, mentioned earlier). He responded, "A lot," and went on to state that the energy required for the embryo to divide and the energy necessary for the embryo to implant really are functions of what has been provided by the mitochondria of the follicle. According to Dr. Brown, "To have an effect on the follicle's mitochondria and to impact adhesions and scar tissue, then enough photons need to reach the target tissues, the ovaries and the pelvic cavity." He added that, to date, the current home systems on the market just don't have the ideal wavelength or power to get an adequate dose of light to penetrate deep enough to the deeper tissues to have a therapeutic effect at the level of the mitochondria of the follicles. This is especially the case if the home system is used off the body (not making contact with the skin), which is common for most home systems for safety; the LEDs are too hot to make skin contact. Dr. Brown recommends both professional systems and home systems for patients. They can use their home systems to help with systemic inflammation while also receiving professional photobiomodulation and laser acupuncture treatments two or three times per week to get therapeutic doses of photons into the deep target areas in the pelvic cavity, which is beneficial for optimizing egg quality and uterine receptivity.

Dr. Brown is a leader in incorporating photobiomodulation treatments with his fertility patients and is hopeful to see laser acupuncture and LLLT used for increasing energy levels (ATP) in the cells, improving blood circulation, stem cell proliferation, the softening of scar tissue, and the reduction of inflammation. These factors are all beneficial to female reproduction in general and to the receptivity of the uterine lining specifically.

On his website, Dr. Brown also states,

Like most discoveries, low level laser therapy (LLLT/photobiomodulation) for fertility was discovered by accident.

Dr. Ohshiro, a medical doctor and pain specialist in Japan, used LLLT to treat pain. He heard back from a 55-year-old menopausal woman who he had treated for back pain that her menses had started again. Months later, another woman in menopause came in for back pain, received laser therapy, and her cycle returned as well.

Since the initial discovery by Dr. Ohshiro, there have been several clinical studies in Japan and elsewhere to explore the potential of low-level laser therapy to help with infertility and other issues including PCOS, uterine receptivity, sperm motility, endometriosis, embryo quality as well as IVF acupuncture on the day of transfer to increase implantation rates.

Studies show that the mitochondria of older eggs are capable of producing significantly less ATP, which is the source of cellular energy. This has a significant impact on fertility, as the rate of division and successful implantation of embryos has more to do with how much energy (ATP) than with maternal age per se. Consequently, the capacity of the cold laser to improve the ATP production of eggs has a potentially dramatic effect on their viability.

Furthermore, it is known that older follicles have fewer defenses against cellular damage caused by oxidative stress, and that this is related to poorer IVF outcomes. Studies suggest that LLLT treatment could also help with this condition, along with other complications, which impede fertility later in life.

The primary takeaway from this chapter is that if the body isn't effectively making ATP, it will know that there is not enough energy to support growing a fetus.

Now, to get deeeeep into lesser known and very technical information on antioxidants, refer to Appendix 11A. This is where the appendix gets thick, and it is for health-care professionals and MegaNerds only! I discuss things like NADPH, the NOX gene, and glutamate as an excitatory and inflammatory compound, along with glutamate/GABA balance, Nrf2, autophagy, NAD+ and the SIRT (sirtuin) genes, and nitric oxide. I also include action steps in Appendix 11A.

REFERENCES

Babayev, Elnur, and Emre Seli. 2015. "Oocyte mitochondrial function and reproduction." *Current Opinion in Obstetrics & Gynecology* 27, no. 3, 175.

Ben-Meir, Assaf, Eliezer Burstein, Aluet Borrego-Alvarez, Jasmine Chong, Ellen Wong, Tetyana Yavorska, Taline Naranian, et al. 2015. "Coenzyme Q10 restores oocyte mitochondrial function and fertility during reproductive aging." *Aging Cell* 14, no. 5, 887–895.

Bertoldo, Michael J., Dave R. Listijono, Wing-Hong Jonathan Ho, Angelique H. Riepsamen, Dale M. Goss, Dulama Richani, Xing L. Jin, et al. 2020. "NAD+ repletion rescues female fertility during reproductive aging." *Cell Reports* 30, no. 6, 1670–1681.

Depeint, Flore, W. Robert Bruce, Nandita Shangari, Rhea Mehta, and Peter J. O'Brien. 2006. "Mitochondrial function and toxicity: role of the B vitamin family on mitochondrial energy metabolism." *Chemico-Biological Interactions* 163, no. 1–2, 94–112.

Haskett, Dorothy R. 2014. "Mitochondrial DNA (mtDNA)." *Embryo Project Encyclopedia*, December 19. https://embryo.asu.edu/pages/mitochondrial-dna-mtdna.

Miao, Yilong, Zhaokang Cui, Qian Gao, Rong Rui, and Bo Xiong. 2020. "Nicotinamide mononucleotide supplementation reverses the declining quality of maternally aged oocytes." *Cell Reports* 32, no. 5, 107987.

Naviaux, Robert K. 2020. "Perspective: cell danger response biology – the new science that connects environmental health with mitochondria and the rising tide of chronic illness." *Mitochondrion* 51, 40–45.

Pizzorno, Joseph. 2014. "Mitochondria – fundamental to life and health." *Integrative Medicine: A Clinician's Journal* 13, no. 2, 8.

Reader, Karen L., Jo-Ann L. Stanton, and Jennifer L. Juengel. 2017. "The role of oocyte organelles in determining developmental competence." *Biology* 6, no. 3, 35.

Saihara, Kazuhiro, Ryosuke Kamikubo, Kazuto Ikemoto, Koji Uchida, and Mitsugu Akagawa. 2017. "Pyrroloquinoline quinone, a redox-active o-quinone, stimulates mitochondrial biogenesis by activating the SIRT1/PGC-1α signaling pathway." *Biochemistry* 56, no. 50, 6615–6625.

Tatone, Carla, Giovanna Di Emidio, Maurizio Vitti, Michela Di Carlo, Silvano Santini, Anna Maria D'Alessandro, Stefano Falone, and Fernanda Amicarelli. 2015. "Sirtuin functions in female fertility: possible role in oxidative stress and aging." *Oxidative Medicine and Cellular Longevity* 2015.

Truong, T., and D. K. Gardner. 2017. "Antioxidants improve IVF outcome and subsequent embryo development in the mouse." *Human Reproduction* 32, no. 12, 2404–2413.

12 Toxins, Toxins, Everywhere: Prioritize Avoiding Toxins!

This is a chapter title that gets an exclamation point because I want to emphasize that this is more important than most people may think.

In the current state of our environment, we get exposed to more toxins in one day than our ancestors of a thousand years ago got in their entire lifetimes. I'm sure that many people who know me roll their eyes at me for being "extra" in my vigilance regarding my avoidance of toxins. What they don't know is that there are tons of peer reviewed journals from the National Library of Medicine that link miscarriage and infertility (and a plethora of other health conditions) to toxin exposure. To quote a site (Sinclair and Pressinger n.d.) that summarizes and references a large number of these medical journal studies,

> Miscarriage and infertility was found to increase from pesticides in food, chemicals in cosmetics, cigarettes, synthetic building materials, alcohol, coffee, food additives, water bottle chemicals, MSG, aspartame, NutraSweet, job occupations, chemicals in air fresheners, vehicle exhaust, detergents, fabric softener, disinfectants, perfumes & more.
>
> Topics discussed also include how these consumer chemicals cause miscarriage and infertility – including research showing lower quality of egg development during the first half of a women's 28-day cycle, damage to the 65-day sperm development process, ability of some chemicals to mimic natural hormones in the body, and the ability for many chemicals to increase autoimmunity against eggs, sperm and fetus.

This research review site also states,

> The same environmental circumstances responsible for infertility and miscarriage can also increase the risk of having a child with mental retardation, learning disabilities or behavior problems (such as ADD).
>
> This is based on the premise that avoidance of these circumstances will also increase the genetic integrity of the child, thereby encouraging maximum gene expression related to all aspects of human behavior from personality – to talent – to academic potential.
>
> Along with this, levels of the common food pesticide DDE were found to impair the oocyte maturation process. For example, DDE was found in the follicle fluid surrounding the egg at levels approximately 1/3rd that of what is in the person's blood. This would suggest that simply eating "organic food"

DOI: 10.1201/b23201-14

would significantly increase the likelihood of achieving a successful pregnancy and higher genetic integrity as studies by the Centers for Disease Control have shown dramatic reductions in blood levels of pesticides 3 days after switching to an all organic food diet.

These findings clearly demonstrate how strict avoidance of specific synthetic chemicals can prevent infertility and miscarriage in many cases.

So basically, if those eye-rollers knew this, as well as all the ways our antioxidant and detoxification pathways can become compromised, they might become a bit more vigilant as well.

Our poor livers were not designed to handle all this work.

12.1 TOXINS AND HORMONES

Regarding hormones, this is how it was for ages: The body makes hormones. The hormones travel to where they need to go, fit into cell receptors (just as a key fits into the right keyhole), which signals the cell to do something. The "used" hormone gets sent to the liver to be metabolized and sends it on its way to the gut, to then get eliminated from the body in the stool.

But this is how it is now: When we have xenoestrogens ("foreign estrogens" that are hormone mimickers that come from things like plastics, receipt paper, pesticides, and the ingredients in cosmetics and body care products) coming into the body, as they do in so many ways these days, they fit into the cell receptors, but instead of signaling the cell to do something, it's like putting superglue into the keyhole. The cell is not given a proper signal to do its thing, so the xenoestrogens cannot be properly metabolized. This creates "feedback" signaling impairments and a buildup of both the xenoestrogens and endogenously produced (made by the body) estrogens, which leads to the estrogen dominance that is the cause of many of the "period problems" and reproductive difficulties women experience these days.

To add insult to injury, the liver prioritizes clearing out the foreign estrogens, so it puts the endogenously produced estrogens on the back burner, which also results in build-up and creates imbalance.

If we can limit the amount of toxins that our lovely livers have to process, that leaves more energy for the liver to do what it was designed to do, including metabolizing the hormones our bodies produce.

12.2 TOXINS AND MITOCHONDRIAL ENERGY PRODUCTION (OR LACK THEREOF)

In previous chapters, I wrote about the mitochondria and how important they are for energy (ATP) production and mating ability. If the body is not able to make ATP efficiently, or if it gets the memo that there is danger/stress and it needs to conserve its energetic resources, it will shut down reproductive capacities.

That same article I referenced in Chapter 11 (Naviaux 2020) goes on to state that numerous studies now report the presence of dozens to hundreds of manmade chemicals and pollutants in placentas and umbilical cord blood and that fewer than 5% of these chemicals have been tested for developmental toxicity. Naviaux's article mentions that a study conducted by the Environmental Working Group in 2005 found that the umbilical cord blood of newborn babies in the United States already contained an average of 287 pesticides, pollutants, and other environmental chemicals. This demonstrates that a child is born having inherited not only their parents' genes but also some of their chemical exposures. There is a documentary called "Ten Americans" that details this study and its findings.

Naviaux continues with discussing how many of these chemicals bioaccumulate and are biomagnified in fat, bone, and reproductive organs, accumulating over years of exposure to levels that can be hundreds of times higher than the concentration in any given environmental source of air, water, or food.

He does state that many banned pesticides like DDT and industrial chemicals like PCBs can still be found in people decades later; however, what he does not mention is that those chemicals are still being produced and used in other countries. Even though DDT was banned in the US decades ago, we import food from countries that still use it.

If that isn't horrifying enough, here's where Naviaux hammers the nail that seals the coffin:

> If a child is born today with a burden of 300 manmade chemicals, in 25 years that child will add to their inherited burden by accumulating new toxic chemicals from their environment as they grow to reproductive maturity. As adults, they will then pass on a new sample of both their inherited and their newly accumulated environmental chemicals to their children. If a net increase of 50 environmental pollutants occurs in the umbilical cord blood with each generation, and is added to the current number of 300, the toxic chemicals passed on to our children will soon have more devastating effects on human health than any mutation in DNA, leading to escalating infertility rates, miscarriages, childhood and adult chronic disease.

This is why we need to make sure we do our best to limit the amount of toxins we are exposed to and also to ensure that our detoxification pathways receive routine maintenance and tender loving care. It's not just for us or our ability to "have a baby" but for generations down the line.

Today, even the most remote parts of the earth are soiled with toxins, whether on the land, in the water, or in the air. I've just detailed studies that show how toxins affect and impair fertility, and in the next chapter, I share how to support their proper detoxification with precision. But before I do that, I want to share the most common and ubiquitous sources of toxins and how to avoid or minimize them. It is way easier and more beneficial to avoid the toxins than it is to detoxify them.

12.3 PLASTICS

There is an enormous amount of ranting about plastic's effects on the environment that I could write, but I'll keep it to myself and only discuss a few of its impacts on health.

First of all, do not think that "BPA-free" plastics are a safer alternative. Bisphenol A (BPA) is widely known to be an endocrine system disruptor that is also linked with

- Infertility
- Recurrent miscarriages (Sugiura-Ogasawara et al. 2005)
- Decreased number of eggs retrieved during IVF
- Implantation failure (Ehrlich et al. 2012)
- Chromosomal abnormalities (Caserta et al. 2014)
- PCOS (Tarantino et al. 2013; Kandaraki et al. 2011)

And outside of affecting reproduction:

- Autoimmunity to brain and nerve tissue (Kharrazian and Vojdani 2017)
- Cardiovascular disease
- Diabetes
- Epigenetic changes that alter the gene expression and can be passed to offspring

Because the public is now aware of these connections, the plastics industry created other bisphenols, like BPS, but studies are showing that BPS exerts similar endocrine-disrupting characteristics. These are similar in structure molecularly, with only slight differences. Plastics and many toxins are xenoestrogens that act as hormone mimickers, as I have mentioned. Plus, plastic is just terrible for the earth and all its creatures. It is contaminating our water, making us estrogenic. Fish are contaminated with it to the point that certain species of fish and amphibians have been found to have female eggs within male testes. *Whaaaat?*

Nano-size plastics are a very real problem and are getting into our bodies on a daily basis. They are bioaccumulating on the earth and in our bodies. Various news sites have reported on a study by the World Wide Fund for Nature that we likely swallow a credit card size's worth of plastic *each week*. For reference, 100% of waterway samples in Pennsylvania (my home state) tested positive for microplastics. We must be certain not only to use high-quality water filtration but also to reduce the amount of plastic we consume (including synthetic fabrics from blankets and clothes like yoga pants and fleece that shed microplastics down the drain each time they are laundered) if we want to try to curb this rampant infestation of plastic into our bodies and the bodies of the animals we consume.

So please don't go thinking that your exposure to plastic isn't contributing to your hormonal imbalance in any way.

In fact, various types of microplastics have been found in human placentas (Ragusa et al. 2021). And polystyrene nanoparticles were also observed in the placenta and in fetal liver, lungs, heart, kidney, and brain, suggesting maternal lung-to-fetal-tissue nanoparticle translocation in late-stage pregnancy (Fournier et al. 2020).

Action Steps

- Don't buy plastic water bottles. Period. Filter and refill. Look into glass and stainless steel. Refer to the resources section for water filtration options.

- Do not touch receipt paper if you don't have to. BPA is what makes receipt paper shiny and smooth.
- Get the plastic out of your house (like food and beverage containers) and try to minimize foods packaged in plastic. If you have children, don't get them plastic teething toys, eating utensils, or plates/bowls.

12.4 PESTICIDES

If the earth's soil, air, and water are toxic, we living beings are toxic. There are about a gazillion papers on pesticides and reproductive health and the damage that they cause.

Pesticides are designed to harm and kill living creatures. You may be thinking, "Yeah, but those doses are so tiny; they don't affect us."

If we are getting small, repeated exposures daily, filling our buckets faster than our poor livers can clear (and some people have more of a genetic predisposition for sub-optimal clearing of pesticides, like with PON1 genetic variants), then our buckets get filled even more quickly with incessant small doses that create a cumulative effect. Anything non-organic is likely cultivated with chemical fertilizers and sprayed with pesticides, as well as herbicides, rodenticides, and/or fungicides.

I am both surprised and thankful that the USDA has a website called WhatsOnMy-Food.org. It details the data of the USDA Pesticide Data Program, which is a pesticide residue–monitoring program that tested over 100 different foods for a couple of hundred different pesticides. They then categorized the pesticides that were found on any given food into known or probable carcinogens, hormone disruptors, neurotoxins, developmental or reproductive toxins, and/or toxins to honeybees and how many of them were found on each particular food.

I want to make an important point that when people think of avoiding pesticides and buying organic, they usually only think about produce. It is very important to buy organic meat and dairy products (if you eat them) as well. Toxins are lipophilic, which means they have an affinity for fat, and so they accumulate in fat cells. So, when animals are fed grains that are genetically modified or sprayed with chemicals or are given pharmaceuticals like hormones and antibiotics, those chemicals accumulate in their fat, and we eat them. Also, the cotton sheets we sleep on and the cotton feminine products we use against our "lady parts" are heavily sprayed with pesticides. Cotton is one of the top four GMO crops and is considered the dirtiest because it is the most heavily sprayed. Because we don't eat cotton, it is often not considered in the conversation about buying organic.

ACTION STEPS

- Buy organic for what your budget will allow, especially for the foods that you consume the most often. Organic farming is good for us, our farmers, and our earth. Even better, buy organic from local farms.
- Discussed more in depth in the next action steps for heavy metals, one simple yet very effective way to eliminate toxins like pesticides and herbicides from your body is through sweating. Get yourself sweating regularly. Check the resources section for my recommendation on an affordable portable sauna.

12.5 HEAVY METALS

Setting: Earth, 21st century. There are heavy metals everywhere in our food, water, and air. The body has a hard time clearing them, so unless they are proactively detoxified, they bioaccumulate. This basically means they get "swept under the rug" and stored away in the body (for example, in the bones, fat tissue, and glands, which affect hormonal balance). But just because they are hidden away does not mean that they are not doing damage to the body.

Heavy metals increase the body's susceptibility to autoimmune conditions, and they disrupt metabolic pathways and cellular processes, affecting mitochondrial energy production (ATP) in the body. And I'm sure you know by now that the body needs to know that energy production is good before it can feel it is a safe time to procreate.

There are different types of testing that can be done to detect heavy metals in the body, such as blood, urine, and hair. Each testing method has its advantages and disadvantages. With regard to reproduction, lead, mercury, and cadmium are toxicants that cross the placenta and accumulate in fetal tissues. Prenatal exposure to mercury and lead poses a health threat, particularly to the developing brain. Fetal exposures to lead and cadmium correlate with reduced birth weight and birth size (Gundacker and Hengstschläger 2012).

ACTION STEPS

Note: Heavy metal detoxification can be very dangerous, and I do not recommend you attempt it without guidance from a knowledgeable practitioner, especially if you are trying to conceive. I recommend if someone is detoxifying metals, or any form of detox for that matter, that they do it four to six months before trying to conceive. This is because stirring up toxins in the body will make them more likely to pass to the unborn child. I also do not recommend doing any type of detoxification while pregnant or breastfeeding, as toxins also pass through the placenta and breast milk.

- Sweating. Our ancient ancestors knew that sweating offered benefits of relaxation, purification, and healing. Sweating is one of the easiest ways to help the body get rid of toxins and heavy metals like lead, cadmium, mercury (Sears et al. 2012), and hexavalent chromium (the "Erin Brockovich toxin"). Studies have shown that more toxins are excreted in sweat than in urine or blood plasma. Anything that makes you sweat will do the trick, although far-infrared (FIR) saunas move the needle the most. Sweating releases metabolic waste, viruses (your body sweats to break a fever), and various toxins (including BPA and glyphosate, the stated active ingredient in RoundUp). FIR energy increases mitochondrial energy production (which fertility is dependent on) and promotes better blood circulation, so nutrients can be carried into cells and metabolic waste and toxins can be carried out of cells more efficiently. There are many more benefits of FIR sauna therapy, but I wanted to highlight the benefits of sweating itself. I absolutely love my sauna. It is my calm space, my healing space, and the place where I am most likely to do some form of meditation. Use caution and start slowly (not doing saunas that are very hot or very long) if you are someone that has a "sensitive body constitution" or a history of chronic illness. Avoid if there is any possibility of pregnancy. Check the resources section for my recommendations on an affordable portable sauna.

- Binders. Completely different from herbs that encourage bowel evacuation, binders are substances that "bind" to toxins for safe escort out of the body. They prevent "enterohepatic recirculation," which happens when toxins are not bound for excretion via the GI tract, so they stay in circulation, and the liver continually has to try to process them. There are various binders, each having its own affinity for binding specific toxins, from metals to biotoxins (like mycotoxins). For example, silica is good for detoxifying aluminum, and modified citrus pectin has shown to be effective for arsenic, cadmium, and lead. One of my favorite binders is G.I. Detox[1] because it contains an array of binders to cover many bases.
- Remineralize to displace metals. Deficiencies in essential minerals predispose a greater potential for toxic heavy metal retention. Certain minerals have affinities for specific tissues and organs. Because minerals and metals can occupy the same enzyme binding sites, if minerals are available, the body will be able to displace the metal and push it out. If there are not enough minerals available, the body will use the metals instead. This is why cadmium can get into the bones and displace zinc, affecting bone strength.
- Avoid dental procedures that put metal into the mouth and teeth, if possible.
- Avoid seafoods that are high in metals, industrial waste, pesticides (from runoff), and PCBs. The larger and older the fish, the more time it has had to accumulate these toxins. Also, avoid freshwater fish from polluted rivers and lakes. Also, when trying to conceive, I recommend avoiding shellfish altogether.
- Eat small fish with shorter lifespans, such as sardines, anchovies, and wild salmon.
- Avoid aluminum deodorants.

12.6 MOLD EXPOSURE AND MYCOTOXINS

This topic was discussed in Chapter 7, but because it impacts reproduction on numerous levels, I wanted to address this (bio)toxin again.

Many species of mold have effects on our health, including fertility and pregnancy outcomes (Kyei et al. 2020). Mold puts the body into a state of alarm. It damages mitochondrial health, which I've mentioned has everything to do with the body's mating ability.

Mold affects hormone levels. Mold activates mast cells, causing them to be "trigger happy." It causes a histamine response, which I discuss in depth in Chapter 16. Remember that histamine and estrogen feed each other, so the mold that activates mast cells to release histamine can cause an elevation in estrogen.

Mycotoxins stimulate NOX (detailed in Chapter 11 appendix), which inhibits your NADPH, a super important molecule that many essential processes in the body are dependent on, like proper glutathione recycling for detoxification. So, mycotoxins essentially inhibit their own detoxification. Interestingly, many types of mold and mycotoxins are detoxified through the liver's glucuronidation pathway (read about this in Chapter 13), which is also a major player in hormonal health. If mycotoxins are clogging up the glucuronidation pathway, hormones will not be able to get effectively cleared. Comparatively, the methylation pathway does not detoxify nearly as many mycotoxins as the glucuronidation pathway. This reiterates a major point of this book: that MTHFR and the methylation pathway are not the only culprits in miscarriages and poor detoxification ability.

Previous exposures to mold can create a significant body burden. If you have lived or worked in a place that had visible mold (but remember, most mycotoxins are not visible), smelled musty, or had sort of water damage (leaks, floods, etc.), that exposure could have allowed mycotoxins to colonize in your body. Certain forms of colonized mold produce oxalates, and if you read Chapter 9 on oxalates, you know how they affect hormones and, therefore, could impact reproductive capacity.

Mold exposure, especially when it colonizes in the body and forms mycotoxins, is such an insidious problem that is not to be taken lightly. I tell my clients that if they have to stop seeing me and stop their personalized protocols in order to be able to deal with remediating the mold in their home (or work, school, etc.), then I fully support that because no matter how fantastically their protocol works, it won't help long term if the source of the problem is not taken care of.

I wrote the action steps to take for mold and mycotoxins in Chapter 7, so refer back to that if you suspect past or current mold exposure could be affecting your health or fertility.

12.7 INDOOR AIR QUALITY

It has been said that our indoor air quality is worse than outdoor air quality these days. With all the housecleaning products, varnishes, carpet/rugs, furniture, paint, air "fresheners," flame retardants, and VOCs in our house today, along with the mold and dust, I'm not surprised.

ACTION STEPS

- Air purifier. I recommend using an air purifier in rooms that you frequent, even if it means moving it to your bedroom at night and home office during the day, for example. Get the best purifier you can afford.
- Dehumidifier. I recommend using a dehumidifier since mold has a difficult time growing in humidity below 60%. If you live in a house with a basement, I think it is safe to say that a dehumidifier is a must.

12.8 BODY CARE PRODUCTS

It has been estimated that a woman is exposed to well over 100 different chemicals before she even leaves her house in the morning. These include nail polish, lotions, hair care products, perfumes, deodorant, feminine care products (yes, there are chemicals in those[2]), and *all* the makeup things. Many of these cosmetic products and ingredients do not need FDA premarket approval, with the exception of color additives, (FDA n.d.) and many that are all too common in the US, like parabens, have actually been banned in Europe.

ACTION STEPS

- Avoid phthalates. Phthalates, often found with parabens, are chemicals that make these products get sudsy and smell good. High levels of phthalates have been shown to lower IVF success rates because they are endocrine disruptors that interfere with the body's ability to metabolize estrogen.
- Refer to the Environmental Working Group's Skin Deep database at ewg. org – I love this resource and recommend it to my clients all the time. It reviews hazardous ingredients for over 70,000 cosmetics and body care products and the ingredients they contain. You can look up a product you use and see its overall rating from one to eight (one being the cleanest and safest). Each ingredient in the product is then reviewed and rated from one to eight. These ratings are given after much scrutiny by toxicologists, chemists, and epidemiologists.
- Download the DetoxMe app by the Silent Spring Institute. It gives easy-to-follow recommendations in such a fun way, you can almost make a game out of it!

In summary, our bodies were not designed to be able to handle so many of these things, especially when bombarded by them all at once, every day, all day long. If our bodies can't properly metabolize them, they act as biochemical and metabolic wrenches in our systems.

Our poor livers, lymphatic systems, and fat cells are trying desperately to process, transport, or store away toxins at a rate they can't keep up with.

Now, dear reader, I'm sure you're ready to move on to liver detoxification processes after all that. Detoxification ability may be more important than nourishment these days.

NOTES

1 www.amazon.com/dp/B00GOFY02Y?tag=squarespace0a-20&linkCode=osi&th=1&psc=1.
2 www.jaclyndowns.com/blog/2016/1/12/natural-selection-of-feminine-products.

REFERENCES

Caserta, Donatella, Noemi Di Segni, Maddalena Mallozzi, Valentina Giovanale, Alberto Mantovani, Roberto Marci, and Massimo Moscarini. 2014. "Bisphenol A and the female reproductive tract: an overview of recent laboratory evidence and epidemiological studies." *Reproductive Biology and Endocrinology* 12, no. 1, 1–10.

Ehrlich, Shelley, Paige L. Williams, Stacey A. Missmer, Jodi A. Flaws, Katharine F. Berry, Antonia M. Calafat, Xiaoyun Ye, John C. Petrozza, Diane Wright, and Russ Hauser. 2012. "Urinary bisphenol A concentrations and implantation failure among women undergoing in vitro fertilization." *Environmental Health Perspectives* 120, no. 7, 978–983.

FDA. n.d. *FDA authority over cosmetics: how cosmetics are not FDA-approved, but are FDA-regulated.* www.fda.gov/cosmetics/cosmetics-laws-regulations/fda-authority-over-cosmetics-how-cosmetics-are-not-fda-approved-are-fda-regulated#Does_FDA_approve.

Fournier, Sara B., Jeanine N. D'Errico, Derek S. Adler, Stamatina Kollontzi, Michael J. Goedken, Laura Fabris, Edward J. Yurkow, and Phoebe A. Stapleton. 2020. "Nanopolystyrene translocation and fetal deposition after acute lung exposure during late-stage pregnancy." *Particle and Fibre Toxicology* 17, no. 1, 1–11.

Gundacker, Claudia, and Markus Hengstschläger. 2012. "The role of the placenta in fetal exposure to heavy metals." *Wiener Medizinische Wochenschrift* 162, no. 9, 201–206.

Kandaraki, Eleni, Antonis Chatzigeorgiou, Sarantis Livadas, Eleni Palioura, Frangiscos Economou, Michael Koutsilieris, Sotiria Palimeri, Dimitrios Panidis, and Evanthia Diamanti-Kandarakis. 2011. "Endocrine disruptors and polycystic ovary syndrome (PCOS): elevated serum levels of bisphenol A in women with PCOS." *The Journal of Clinical Endocrinology & Metabolism* 96, no. 3, E480–E484.

Kharrazian, Datis, and Aristo Vojdani. 2017. "Correlation between antibodies to bisphenol A, its target enzyme protein disulfide isomerase and antibodies to neuron-specific antigens." *Journal of Applied Toxicology* 37, no. 4, 479–484.

Kyei, Nicholas N. A., Daniel Boakye, and Sabine Gabrysch. 2020. "Maternal mycotoxin exposure and adverse pregnancy outcomes: a systematic review." *Mycotoxin Research* 36, no. 2, 243–255.

Naviaux, Robert K. 2020. "Perspective: cell danger response biology – The new science that connects environmental health with mitochondria and the rising tide of chronic illness." *Mitochondrion* 51, 40–45.

Ragusa, Antonio, Alessandro Svelato, Criselda Santacroce, Piera Catalano, Valentina Notarstefano, Oliana Carnevali, Fabrizio Papa, et al. 2021. "Plasticenta: first evidence of microplastics in human placenta." *Environment International* 146, 106274.3

Sears, Margaret E., Kathleen J. Kerr, and Riina I. Bray. 2012. "Arsenic, cadmium, lead, and mercury in sweat: a systematic review." *Journal of Environmental and Public Health* 2012.

Sinclair, Wayne, and Richard W. Pressinger. n.d. *Environmental causes of infertility.* www.chem-tox.com/infertility/.

Sugiura-Ogasawara, Mayumi, Yasuhiko Ozaki, Shin-ichi Sonta, Tsunehisa Makino, and Kaoru Suzumori. 2005. "Exposure to bisphenol A is associated with recurrent miscarriage." *Human Reproduction* 20, no. 8, 2325–2329.

Tarantino, Giovanni, Rossella Valentino, Carolina Di Somma, Vittoria D'Esposito, Federica Passaretti, Genoveffa Pizza, Valentina Brancato, et al. 2013. "Bisphenol A in polycystic ovary syndrome and its association with liver – spleen axis." *Clinical Endocrinology* 78, no. 3, 447–453.

13 Optimize Your Liver Detoxification Pathways and Detoxify with Precision

If your liver isn't detoxifying, you will have inflammation, and if you have inflammation, your liver won't be detoxifying. When detoxification demands become overburdening, liver function can become significantly impaired. Liver detoxification requires amino acids, vitamins, and minerals. I do not recommend that someone embark on a major cleanse or detox until they have bolstered their body with supportive nutrients, and the body is robust enough to withstand the physical stress that detox may cause. Also, a clinical pearl that I can't emphasize enough is that you must always make sure that elimination channels are open before doing any detoxification. Keep in mind that "metabolism" essentially is the cellular ability to make energy and manage it so that the cells have the strength to eliminate toxins; toxin removal should simply be a competent step in the natural sequence of cellular events. Nourishing and restoring that metabolic competence and capability will make any detox program more effective and less symptomatically severe.

13.1 DRAINAGE BEFORE DETOXIFICATION

One gentle way to begin detoxification is through drainage, which is opening up the dctoxification pathways so that thcy can effectively eliminate toxins. You want to make sure you're pooping a minimum of once per day. If you are not, then toxins are building up, and that should be the first place to start; otherwise, where will the toxins you release during detoxification go if you aren't getting them out of your body? They will get reabsorbed, a process called enterohepatic circulation. Supporting drainage will also help prevent hardcore die-off symptoms during detoxification. A few basic ways to support drainage are deep breathing, exercise/moving your body lovingly, dry brushing, rebounding, ensuring proper water intake, sweating, massage, and using herbs like burdock and astragalus. Also refer to the resources section of this book for recommendations on a drainage kit that helps open detox pathways.

When talking about detoxification and hormone metabolism, I want to distinguish between phase 1 and phase 2 liver detoxification. Many, if not most, toxins are fat soluble (Figure 13.1). As I stated in Chapter 4, phase 1 detox is when the liver takes fat-soluble compounds and transforms them into reactive intermediates with the help of the cytochrome P450 mono-oxygenase (CYP) enzymes (made by an array of CYP genes). These intermediary metabolites are often more toxic than the original toxin!

DOI: 10.1201/b23201-15

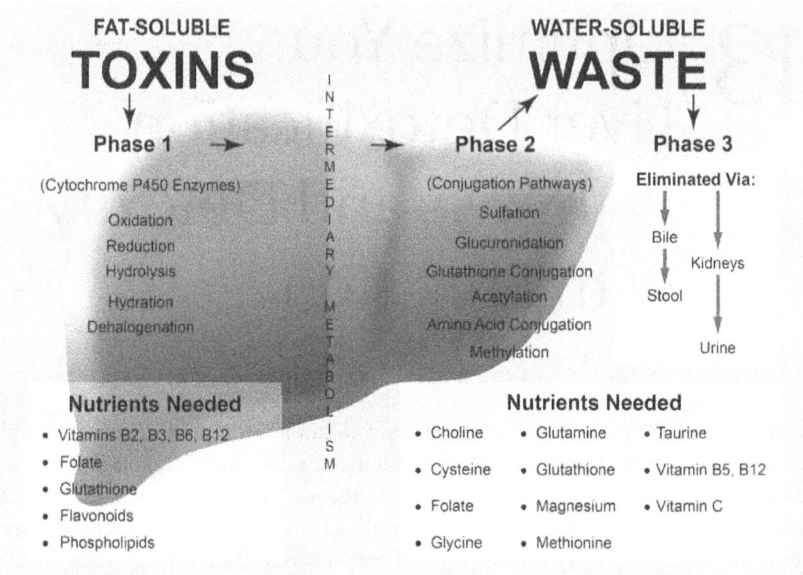

FIGURE 13.1 Three phases of liver detoxification and the nutrients involved.

We must make sure that phase 2 can effectively follow phase 1. With no exaggeration, the "crummier" the food habits and lifestyle are, the greater the demands and strain on the liver will be and the quicker the liver will "give out" in its ability to detoxify the blood.

For a deep dive into phase 1 and 2 liver detoxification and related pathways and genes, refer to Appendix 13A.

Think of it like the trash in your house. You can collect the trash from bins in each room throughout the house, and you can put the trash from those bins into a big garbage bag to go out, but if the front door won't open so that the trash can actually be taken out of the house, things will quickly get backed up. And that's just for everyday life, not major spring cleaning. Before embarking on a detox, you want to ensure that waste removal is happening before doing a major cleaning. This means that first, the gut must be working optimally with no constipation, or what is considered phase 3 detox. The bowels (and kidneys for that matter) have to be working well to be able to handle the increased toxic load when the liver starts "cleaning house." Next, bile must be moving well to transport the toxins from the liver to the bowels to be excreted (what I consider phase 2.5 and phase 3). We must also ensure that phase 2 is up to snuff before supporting phase 1.

Even though liver detoxification phases are ordered in the way that toxins are metabolized and excreted from the body, when embarking on a detox or cleanse, you want to take a "bottom-up" approach.

It is important to note that even if people with phase 2 detox issues don't have fertility challenges, the toxins that their bodies have difficulty eliminating will absolutely be shared with their babies in utero and through the breast milk. This is why

I highly recommend that anyone even considering an inkling of the possibility of having children someday work proactively on getting the toxins out, ideally at least a minimum of six months prior to conceiving.

This chapter is for my hardcore nerds who really want to dig deep into the subject of detoxification and the genes relating to each pathway. I also tie this information to how fertility may be affected. Because of this, much of the content is going to be in Appendix 13, which gets into the genes and the nitty gritty of the phase 2 detoxification pathways sulfation/sulfonation, glucuronidation, glutathione conjugation, and acetylation. Methylation was discussed in Chapter 4. I provide some interesting and basic tidbits here, but the more technical "whys" and "hows" are detailed in Appendix 13.

13.2 SULFATION IS CRITICAL FOR HORMONAL HEALTH

The body requires sulfates to inactivate hormones like estrone and estradiol, so people with low sulfate levels from oxalate issues, genetic predisposition, and/or low intake of sulfur-rich foods very often have hormonal imbalance, which often presents with endometriosis, fibroids, and/or PCOS, which can lead to reproductive issues.

Sulfate is needed for hormone synthesis. Cholesterol is the mother of all reproductive and stress hormones. Hormone signaling is a slow process, and if we can't sulfate hormones, they swing wildly or are greatly depleted across the board, and cholesterol can do the same thing if not sulfated properly. If we don't have good levels of sulfate, then cholesterol levels won't be good, so neither will bile, which will result in fat malabsorption, and that will lead to hormone imbalance since we need fats to make hormones. Refer back to Chapter 10 on the topic of fat malabsorption issues.

13.3 SULFATION ABILITY IMPACTS THYROID HORMONES

We have sulfate transporters all over the body, and almost all systems utilize sulfur compounds in one way or another. Thyroid hormones are not any different. Sulfation plays a role in the inactivation of thyroid hormones, and research has discussed the importance of thyroid hormone sulfation during fetal development.

13.4 VITAMIN D LEVELS CAN BE DEFICIENT IF SOMEONE DOESN'T HAVE SULFATE

The sunlight that kisses our skin is dependent on sulfate (in the sulfide form) and nitric oxide (eNOS) to be turned into vitamin D sulfate, which is a water-soluble form of the well-known, fat-soluble vitamin D. Vitamin D sulfate is linked to many genes that we want to have expressed.

Only sulfated vitamin D can travel freely throughout the bloodstream, but the vitamin D found in most supplements is unsulfated. You can't add sulfur to vitamin D after it has become desulfated by biochemical processes. It must start out being sulfated in the skin.

Since vitamin D sulfate is water soluble, it can go through cells into the cytoplasm. Cholesterol is a precursor to vitamin D, as it is a carrier of sulfur. Attachment of sulfate to vitamin D gives it that special access. Cholesterol that is not sulfated cannot travel and is not water soluble. If someone is low in sulfur, could it be that cholesterol rises in a desperate attempt to pick up more sulfur?

Sulfates are essential for health and detoxification. They are required for the production of glutathione, the body's master antioxidant.

Catecholamine (certain neurotransmitters) metabolism also requires sulfation. This includes dopamine and histamine, so you may feel like parts of your brain are on "fast-forward" if they are not being properly metabolized. This can cause feelings of anxiety, easy agitation, mania, insomnia, paranoia, and hyperactivity. This may also be why you feel so chillaxed after an Epsom salt (magnesium sulfate) bath – you're getting the double bonus of magnesium and catecholamine-metabolizing sulfate.

13.5 SULFITE FROM FOODS

Some people are sensitive to sulfites in food. Wine and dried fruit are two commonly known sources. However, a lesser-known tidbit is that non-organic grapes are dunked in sodium metabisulfite, and farm-raised salmon are often preserved with sodium metabisulfite. Read your labels, and know your farmer!

Appendices 13B and 13C discuss the balance between sulfite and sulfate, as well as the SUOX gene that is responsible for converting sulfites into sulfates. Many people blame sulfur intolerance on the SUOX gene, but as you will discover ahead, there are other factors that can be causative.

As I mentioned, factors that can reduce sulfation ability include a low-sulfur diet and administration of xenobiotics such as acetaminophen, which are processed for elimination through sulfation (Hartzell and Seneff 2012).

Sulfate is a necessary and extremely beneficial substance in the body. A fetus depends on the mother for sulfate supply.

ACTION STEPS

- Eat your broccoli and other sulfur-rich cruciferous vegetables. And if you wanna get really down with it, eat broccoli sprouts, but be sure to chew them well.
- Do Epsom salt soaks. Start with a small amount and slowly increase as is tolerated by your body if you think there may be any oxalate issues. You should feel nothing but relaxed after a soak.
- MSM can be used topically or orally, as the 'S' provides the sulfate.
- Molybdenum has been shown to help convert sulfite into sulfate if there are conversion issues.

13.6 GLUCURONIDATION: THE UNSUNG HERO

Glucuronidation is one of the most important and most common phase 2 liver detoxification pathways but is frequently overlooked and underestimated. It is nearly always a route for detoxifying foreign substances. In fact, glucuronidation is involved in 40–75% of xenobiotic elimination, including clinically used drugs. I believe this will become a more frequently discussed topic in the future as its importance becomes more well-known and as our need for proactive detoxification becomes more urgent.

The liver detoxification process of glucuronidation adds a glucuronic acid molecule (a sugar) to a toxin to make it water soluble so it is more easily excreted by the body. Glucuronidation is also a heavy hitter for the clearance of mycotoxins.

This phase 2 pathway actually clears more forms of mycotoxins by far than the other phase 2 pathways. Refer back to the visual diagrams and discussion of mold and mycotoxins in Chapter 7. To listen to a great podcast interview on precision mycotoxin detoxification with a few of my expert colleagues that will school listeners on the glucuronidation pathway, I recommend the BetterHealthGuy.com blogcast episode 122.[1]

In addition to foreign substances, glucuronidation clears endogenous compounds and is the prime phase 2 pathway for bilirubin, estrone, testosterone, progesterone, thyroxine, biotoxins, histamine, and other amines. We will often see estrogen dominance with glucuronidation impairments. The DUTCH test can be a great way to see what is functionally happening with the glucuronidation of hormones. Refer to the Resources section for information about the DUTCH test.

Because it is such a heavy hitter for clearing so many substances, it can, and often does, get overwhelmed. The glucuronidation pathway can get clogged and backed up easily, derailing the hormones.

Clinical pearl: Regarding histamine, even if someone doesn't have any SNPs in histamine-related genes (HNMT, ABP1, MAOB, or the four histamine receptors discussed in Chapter 16), they can still have histamine intolerance issues due to impaired glucuronidation since histamine is cleared via this pathway.

For more information on genes related to the glucuronidation pathway, other functions of it, and factors that inhibit it, refer to Appendix 13D.

Some daily factors that inhibit glucuronidation can include high-carb/low-protein diets; elevated glucose and elevated insulin, independent of each other; reduced caloric intake; depletion of hepatic glycogen stores (endurance athletes); cannabis use; and plastics exposure. The unrelenting amount of plastic and microplastics we encounter and even ingest each week is absolutely placing a heavier burden on our glucuronidation abilities (Luo et al. 2019). Microplastics are now known to have devastating effects on critical periods of development in the neuroendocrine system. They have also been associated with the rising number of cases of a congenital malformation called hypospadias. This is where the opening of the male urethra is on the underside of the penis, instead of at the tip.

ACTION STEPS

There are a few substances that have been shown to boost glucuronidation activity, with my three favorites being on the more inexpensive side.

- Calcium-D-glucarate (CDG) facilitates liver detox, essential for estrogen metabolism. This is especially helpful for women with high estrogen levels, such as those with PCOS or endometriosis.

    o Calcium-D-glucarate may increase glucuronidation and reduce beta-glucuronidase, an enzyme that supports reabsorption of toxic chemicals. CDG can aggressively shift estrogen levels and must be used with caution if you have low estrogen levels. Usually, the higher the beta-glucuronidase levels, the higher the need for CDG.

    o Important note: Before supplementing with something like calcium D-glucarate or DIM for hormonal balance, I strongly encourage hormone testing via the DUTCH test (see Appendix 11) because sometimes symptoms can be the same for high estrogen levels as they are for low.

- Dandelion root may increase UGT enzyme activity in phase 2 glucuronidation. It may also support additional hepatic antioxidant activities by increasing enzyme activity of catalase and various forms of glutathione.
- Nrf2 is critical for UGT enzyme function, which supports the glucuronidation pathway. Astaxanthin induces Nrf2 activity (Niu et al. 2018) and may be an inducer of the UGT glucuronidation enzymes (Gradelet et al. 1996). Astaxanthin also is an important antioxidant carotenoid, as it has been shown to upregulate the antioxidant molecules SOD, NADPH, NQO1, and HMOX (Chen et al. 2018). You will understand how impactful this can be if you read Chapter 11 on antioxidants.
- Green tea, watercress, ellagic acid (chestnuts are a dense source [Ceci et al. 2018]), berries (especially blackberries), pterostilbene, and rosmarinic acid have also been shown to induce and/or support glucuronidation.

When attempting to support glucuronidation, it is imperative to support bile flow first. If you start moving all the toxins from the liver, you better make sure they can be excreted from the body! For supporting bile flow, I like to recommend castor oil packs, coffee enemas, and bitters. I discuss supporting bile flow in Chapter 10 on fat utilization.

13.7 GLUTATHIONE CONJUGATION PATHWAY

Glutathione is both a phase 2 detoxifying compound and an antioxidant. It is used by the liver to detoxify formaldehyde, acetaminophen, specific mycotoxins, benzopyrene, and many other compounds. Glutathione helps maintain cellular redox potential, which means it helps keep antioxidants loaded and ready to fire against inflammation. Glutathione as an antioxidant is involved in protection of proteins, nucleic acid synthesis, and DNA repair.

Glutathione is made up of three amino acids – cysteine, glycine, and glutamic acid. There are quite a few genes involved in both synthesizing glutathione (and its precursors) and in its creation as an antioxidant and detoxifying agent.

I mention a couple of times in this book that glutathione is often incorrectly used in hopes of supporting the clearance of various types of mycotoxins, but the glutathione conjugation pathway has only been shown to effectively clear ochratoxin-A and aflatoxin B1. Although glucuronidation is not the primary clearance pathway for ochratoxin-A and aflatoxin B1, it will pick up the slack when glutathione conjugation is insufficient.

To learn more about these three amino acid components of glutathione, as well as why supplementing with N-acetyl-cysteine may not work or can even backfire in some people, and why glutathione may not be an effective way to clear mycotoxins from the body, refer to Appendix 13E.

13.8 ACTION STEPS: HOW WE SUPPORT GLUTATHIONE AND THE GST GENES

- Luckily, you can almost eat your way out of this! The most significant factors in supporting glutathione are cruciferous vegetables and broccoli sprouts (chewed very well to unlock the enzymes).
- Rosemary and garlic are also fantastic supports for the GST gene/enzyme (Glutathione-S-Transferase) that turns glutathione from an antioxidant to a detoxifying agent.
- Some supplements that can support glutathione levels are alpha lipoic acid, artichoke, curcuminoids, folate, magnesium, silymarin (milk thistle), selenium, and vitamin B6.
- Sometimes it is necessary to use S-acetyl glutathione or liposomal glutathione if there are significant GCLC, GCLM, or GSS variants.
- Also, consider supporting Nrf2 since that can be just as significant as glutathione-related SNPs themselves as many glutathione-related genes require Nrf2 as a cofactor. I discuss Nrf2, its importance, and how to support it in Chapter 11.
- Luckily, a wide array of binders work well for aflatoxin B1. Since different binders have affinities for different toxins (zeolite is well known for heavy metals, activated charcoal for biotoxins, etc.), I really like Biocidin Botanical's G.I. Detox because it is a "gentle" but effective "sponge" to bind toxins for elimination without irritating the gut lining.

13.9 ACETYLATION

Acetylation is a phase 2 liver detoxification pathway that adds an acetyl group to a toxin to make it less reactive and more water soluble for easier elimination. Just like methylation is the exchange of a methyl group, acetylation is the addition of an acetyl group to a compound to catalyze a change. And just like with methylation, acetylation can alter gene expression epigenetically.

Compared to sulfation and glucuronidation, acetylation is modest in terms of the number and variety of substrates, but it remains significant from a toxicological perspective (Jančová and Šiller 2012). The acetylation pathway eliminates lots of different toxins, some of which are aromatic amines, drugs, cigarette smoke, mycotoxins, and certain carcinogens.

13.10 FOR ALL ACETYLATION REACTIONS, WE NEED ADEQUATE ACETYL-COA

Acetyl-CoA is a molecule that participates in many biochemical reactions in protein, carbohydrate, and lipid metabolism. Its primary function is to deliver the acetyl group to the citric acid cycle so that ATP can be made. And I can't repeat this point enough: *If the body can't effectively make ATP, it will shut off mating capabilities.*

Three other important functions that acetyl CoA is used for are:

1. Phase 2 conjugation by acetylation
2. Creating steroidal hormones for lipid synthesis, starting with cholesterol
3. Enabling lipid balance and fluidity in cell membranes, impacting neurological function

To learn more about the genes and cofactors related to acetylation and its importance for hormone health, refer to Appendix 13F.

13.11 ACTION STEPS: BEGINNING TO SUPPORT ACETYLATION

- Carnitine is what shuttles fat into the cell so ATP can be made. Carnitine supports ACAT activity. There is a study showing that carnitine in both forms (acetyl-L-carnitine and L-carnitine) can improve female fertility through their integrated actions on reducing cellular stress, maintaining hormonal balance, and enhancing energy production because of the role it plays in acetylation. These beneficial effects show "great promise in its application as a treatment option for women facing infertility disorders" (Agarwal et al. 2018). Note: The SLC22A5 gene is what makes a protein that shuttles carnitine into the cell. Variants here can hinder this process.
- Calcium pyruvate. This form of calcium bound to pyruvate can support acetyl-CoA production. Carbohydrates are broken down via glycolysis, forming pyruvate. Pyruvate is then transported to the mitochondria to feed into the citric acid cycle.
- Vitamin B5 as pantethine. In appendix 13F, I discussed the importance of pantethine as a primary ingredient for acetyl-CoA to work its magic. Supplementation may be warranted if there are variants in PANK genes or if urinary labs come back low.
- Acetylated supplements provide the body with the acetyl group. These are supplements like S-acetyl-glutathione, N-acetyl-cysteine, acetyl-L-carnitine, and N-acetyl-glucosamine.

13.12 PHASE 2.5 AND PHASE 3 DETOX

Phase 2.5 detox occurs when a toxin has become packaged up and water soluble and is being transported out of the liver and into excretion pathways. Phase 3 detox is the actual elimination from the body via urine sweat, and stool. Many people make the mistake of tackling detoxes by starting with targeting the liver (phase 1 or phase 2), when, as I stated earlier in this chapter, what they really need to do is take a "bottom-up" approach.

The gut needs to be healthy, and the body must be efficiently eliminating waste. We first need to make sure the garbage we are clearing out can be eliminated from the body. If phase 3 is backed up, it will cause a downregulation of phase 2 activity, in which the toxic intermediary metabolites from phase 1 can build up and cause oxidative damage. We must have a healthy functioning gut (discussed in the next chapter) and microbiome for our detoxification capacity to be maximized, minimizing inflammation, which causes chronic issues, especially impaired fertility.

We need liver detoxification to be efficient for many processes that we rely on daily: heavy metal elimination, digestion, immune function, cellular/metabolic function, hormonal harmony, gut integrity, microbial balance. Imbalances in these pathways are huge flags that foundational pillars are out of balance. If we ignore these flags, or let them fly for too long, it is to our own detriment.

ACTION STEPS

- Since the bile is composed primarily of phosphatidylcholine, supplementing with phosphatidylcholine can help improve bile fluidity. Ox bile (not for long-term use unless you've had your gallbladder removed) taken with meals can also be helpful.
- Coffee enemas increase production of glutathione (the "master antioxidant") and are believed to increase dilation of the bile ducts, facilitating toxin excretion. Coffee enemas also benefit the body by stimulating the all-important vagus nerve.
- Colon hydrotherapy is another great option to "clean the pipes." Discuss with your practitioner how often these can be done, as some people tend to overdo things. More is not necessarily better.
- As I already mentioned a few times in this book, bitters (like artichoke and dandelion root) and castor oil packs are good ways to stimulate bile flow, which will assist phase 2.5 and phase 3 detoxification.

NOTE

1   https://betterhealthguy.com/episode122.

REFERENCES

Agarwal, Ashok, Pallav Sengupta, and Damayanthi Durairajanayagam. 2018. "Role of L-carnitine in female infertility." *Reproductive Biology and Endocrinology* 16, no. 1, 1–18.

Ceci, Claudia, Pedro M. Lacal, Lucio Tentori, Maria Gabriella De Martino, Roberto Miano, and Grazia Graziani. 2018. "Experimental evidence of the antitumor, antimetastatic and antiangiogenic activity of ellagic acid." *Nutrients* 10, no. 11, 1756.

Chen, Qing, Jun Tao, and Xi Xie. 2018. "Astaxanthin promotes Nrf2/ARE signaling to inhibit HG-induced renal fibrosis in GMCs." *Marine Drugs* 16, no. 4, 117.

Gradelet, S., Pierre Astorg, Julie Leclerc, J. Chevalier, M. F. Vernevaut, and M-H. Siess. 1996. "Effects of canthaxanthin, astaxanthin, lycopene and lutein on liver xenobiotic-metabolizing enzymes in the rat." *Xenobiotica* 26, no. 1, 49–63.

Hartzell, Samantha, and Stephanie Seneff. 2012. "Impaired sulfate metabolism and epigenetics: is there a link in autism?" *Entropy* 14, no. 10, 1953–1977.

Jančová, Petra, and Michal Šiller. 2012. "Phase II drug metabolism." *Topics on Drug Metabolism* 35–60.

Luo, Ting, Caiyun Wang, Zihong Pan, Cuiyuan Jin, Zhengwei Fu, and Yuanxiang Jin. 2019. "Maternal polystyrene microplastic exposure during gestation and lactation altered metabolic homeostasis in the dams and their F1 and F2 offspring." *Environmental Science & Technology* 53, no. 18, 10978–10992.

Niu, Tingting, Rongrong Xuan, Ligang Jiang, Wei Wu, Zhanghe Zhen, Yuling Song, Lili Hong et al. 2018. "Astaxanthin induces the Nrf2/HO-1 antioxidant pathway in human umbilical vein endothelial cells by generating trace amounts of ROS." *Journal of Agricultural and Food Chemistry* 66, no. 6, 1551–1559.

14 Show Your Guts Some Love

14.1 THE GUT–HORMONE CONNECTION: HOW GUT IMBALANCE LEADS TO INFLAMMATION AND HORMONAL HAVOC

The health of the gut and microbiome are often not a topic of discussion when someone is experiencing impaired fertility. Gut health can be a huge rock that should not be left unturned. So many of my clients experience gut issues, from constipation to diarrhea and from food sensitivities to IBS. Not many people know that leaky gut and dysbiosis can cause premature ovarian failure, diminished ovarian reserve, and other fertility challenges.

There are numerous ways that hormones and fertility can be affected by the impaired functioning of the gut. This includes what is/isn't residing within the gut but also the structural integrity of the gut. Obviously, unwelcome guests in the body, as well as "leaky gut," will disrupt gut functioning and hinder repair and are root causes of so many health conditions.

Intestinal permeability, commonly referred to as "leaky gut," occurs when the gut lining has "holes" in it. Technically, the tight junctions of the lining are stuck open when they are supposed to be closed. This allows incompletely digested food particles into the bloodstream, causing inflammation and immune system reactivity, which can derail fertility. To make matters worse, if the immune system constantly reacts to undigested food proteins in the blood, it will start to identify them as foreign intruders. This is how food sensitivities can begin. If this immune reactivity goes on long enough, the immune system will be amplified to a heightened response and begin to attack anything that resembles the protein structure of the offending food (technically called "molecular mimicry"). When our immune system attacks proteins in our tissues – like the thyroid, for instance – this is an autoimmune response. In the case of the thyroid, the autoimmune condition is Hashimoto's. There is plenty of literature that describes the association between autoimmune conditions and infertility in both sexes (Carp et al. 2012).

Intestinal barrier damage is common and often occurs due to things like alcohol, food allergies, non-steroidal anti-inflammatory drugs (NSAIDs), infection, stress, and toxins like pesticides and heavy metals. Leaky gut has also been tightly associated with poor vagal tone (discussed in Chapter 6).

Since 70–80% of our immune cells are located in the gut, our immune health is greatly dependent on our gut health.

Gut bacteria act as part of the endocrine system. They are involved in converting, activating, and metabolizing different hormones, including thyroid hormones. In fact, there are numerous studies suggesting the interconnectedness of the microbiome

DOI: 10.1201/b23201-16

with fertility-related issues like endometriosis, insulin resistance, thyroid dysfunction, and PCOS.

Dysbiosis occurs when there is an abundance of bad bacteria and not enough of the good. Most of the time, when people talk about dysbiosis, they are referring to the gut microbiota.

Note:

Some people are genetically predisposed to having a microbiome that is less abundant in good bacteria. The FUT2 gene, which codes for the fucosyl-transferase 2 enzyme, plays a role in how diverse and abundant the beneficial bacteria are in the GI tract, especially when it comes to the bifidobacteria. Basically, the FUT2 gene helps create the prebiotics (oligosaccharides called 2'-fucosyllactose) that feed the probiotics in the gut.

But get this – 2'-fucosyllactose is only found in our digestive tract and in breast milk (Lefebvre et al. 2020; Lewis et al. 2015). Women who have a homozygous variant in the FUT2 gene have been found not to secrete 2'-fucosyllactose in their breast milk, whereas women who do not have the SNP do.

We need healthy GI tracts to get rid of estrogen (along with a healthy functioning liver and bile flow, which gets sent to the intestinal tract). Healthy gut bacteria absolutely affect estrogen levels. Dysbiosis can decrease production of the protective estrogen, 2-hydroxyestrone, and increase the production of less desirable estrogens (4-hydroxy and 16-hydroxy). The DUTCH test (see Appendix 11 and the Resources section for more info on this test) can show what your estrogen clearance pathways look like and whether or not you favor the 2-hydroxyestrone pathway.

There are beneficial bacteria in the gut that metabolize estrogens. This aggregate of beneficial bacteria is referred to as the estrobolome. Estrogen metabolism requires a functional estrobolome. If the estrobolome is imbalanced, then a lot of those estrogens get reabsorbed in the gut and back into the bloodstream but aren't usable. This causes problems with hormone balance and the estrogen/progesterone ratio, compounding period problems.

In the previous chapter, in which I discussed glucuronidation, I mentioned beta-glucuronidase, the enzyme that supports reabsorption of toxic chemicals and xenoestrogens. Imbalances in the gut can increase beta-glucuronidase, causing improperly metabolized estrogens and toxins to be recirculated, elevating estrogen levels.

I tell my clients that we can't deeply clean or repair our houses if we have house guests, so we must get rid of them in order to heal the gut. Even if we don't have much in the way of symptoms, our intelligent bodies know there is a stressor causing imbalance, and that causes inflammation. Inflammation will suppress HPA functioning, causing sluggish hormone production. Remember that the thyroid and ovaries are part of the HPA circuit, so their hormonal production will be sluggish as well.

We need healthy gut functioning to be able to absorb the nutrients that are needed for enzymatic reactions to take place. If we aren't absorbing nutrients like iodine, selenium, zinc, and B vitamins (or B vitamin synthesis by various microbiota is impaired), they won't be available to be used as cofactors for these reactions.

Considering this information, it makes sense that dysbiosis of the gut and vaginal microbiomes is a potential indicator of higher rates of failure of IVF (Kong et al. 2020).

Additionally, the best thing we can do for the health of our children, including their long-term health, is to get a healthy gut and vaginal microbiome in place. A mother's gut microbiome influences how her baby's gut microbiome will develop in the first three years of life. Her gut health helps establish theirs!

Action Steps

- Remove sugar, bad fats (trans fats, many seed oils, non-organic animal fats), and foods that may cause you sensitivities. Dairy and gluten are the typical biggies, as are corn, soy, and eggs. These top five most common sensitivities are, not coincidentally, the top five most commonly consumed foods in Western culture. If removing these foods doesn't provide notable relief, you might want to explore diets like AIP, low FODMAP, or GAPS.
- Address gut infections and compromises. Functional lab testing can take the guesswork out but is often not exhaustively conclusive, especially with parasites. Doing a "killing protocol" to remove unwelcome guests (ensuring first that foundational steps are taken so the body is able to withstand the stress of a killing protocol), followed by a rebuilding step to heal the gut lining can often be a big step in improving gut health.
- Diversify and reinoculate the gut with the beneficial bacterial strains it needs. This can be done through fermented foods (if you do not have histamine intolerance; read all about histamine intolerance in chapter 15) or supplementation. Probiotics balance the immune system, fight inflammation, help heal gut issues and skin conditions, and are great for promoting overall digestive wellness. They can even help the body produce certain nutrients like vitamin B12 and vitamin K. I personally love the Mega SporeBiotic supplement for many, if not most, of my clients because the spores get past the stomach acid and arrive in the intestines, where they then become active, as opposed to needing to be specially encapsulated to (hopefully) make it through stomach acid. Rather than merely (and potentially) repopulating the gut with whatever strains are in the bottle, Mega SporeBiotic probiotics help diversify as well as repopulate the microbiome. Improving the health of the gut microbiome will spill over into the vaginal microbiome and help with things like yeast infections and bacterial vaginosis.
- Support the gut with digestive enzymes. Talk with your nutritional practitioner about which kinds would be best for your particular situation.
- Peek at your poo! I can tell a lot about my clients' gut health based on descriptions of their bowel movements. They should happen at least once a day, and they should be well-formed logs that are earthy in color.

You should not see undigested food like bits of lettuce or carrots in them –
corn and seeds are normal. They should not float or leave "skid marks."
(See Chapter 10 on fat utilization if they do.) They should not require lots of
wiping, and they shouldn't be really smelly.

REFERENCES

Carp, Howard J. A., Carlo Selmi, and Yehuda Shoenfeld. 2012. "The autoimmune bases of
    infertility and pregnancy loss." *Journal of Autoimmunity* 38, no. 2–3, J266–J274.
Kong, Yao, Zhaoxia Liu, Qingyao Shang, Yuan Gao, Xia Li, Cihua Zheng, Xiaorong Deng,
    and Tingtao Chen. 2020. "The disordered vaginal microbiota is a potential indicator for
    a higher failure of in vitro fertilization." *Frontiers in Medicine* 7, 217.
Lefebvre, Gregory, Maya Shevlyakova, Aline Charpagne, Julien Marquis, Mandy Vogel,
    Toralf Kirsten, Wieland Kiess, Sean Austin, Norbert Sprenger, and Aristea Binia. 2020.
    "Time of lactation and maternal fucosyltransferase genetic polymorphisms determine
    the variability in human milk oligosaccharides." *Frontiers in Nutrition* 225.
Lewis, Zachery T., Sarah M. Totten, Jennifer T. Smilowitz, Mina Popovic, Evan Parker,
    Danielle G. Lemay, Maxwell L. Van Tassell, et al. 2015. "Maternal fucosyltransferase
    2 status affects the gut bifidobacterial communities of breastfed infants." *Microbiome*
    3, no. 1, 1–21.

15 Histamine Can Affect Reproductive Outcomes

Most people only recognize histamine as it relates to seasonal allergies and allergic reactions (e.g., itchy eyes, runny nose, bronchial constriction). Histamine can cause a lot more problems than just your garden-variety hay fever symptoms, and it absolutely can be a cause of hormonal and reproductive issues.

15.1 WHAT IS HISTAMINE?

Histamine is a compound that is released by mast cells, which are specialized immune cells that are part of our immune system's frontline defense. Mast cells release histamine and dozens of other chemical messengers, called mediators, as an inflammatory response to certain allergens, stressors, or environmental stimuli. Histamine is a signaling molecule that acts as a messenger between cells. It plays many important roles in the body.

Aside from its central role in allergic reactions, histamine also directly influences brain function, blood pressure, sleep, and sexual function. It stimulates gastric acid secretion, helping break down food, and is even involved in pituitary hormone secretion and immunomodulation.

Histamine is contained in almost all tissues in the body, especially the sinuses/nose, skin, and lungs, which are the sites of the most common histamine symptoms. Excess histamine in the body can cause a variety of symptoms including vertigo, headaches/migraines, gastrointestinal issues (like diarrhea and stomach cramping), fatigue, weight gain, and dysmenorrhea (Maintz and Novak 2007), and it can also play a role in pathological processes such as preeclampsia and preterm delivery. In addition to these pregnancy complications, histamine has also been associated with having "significant effects on ovulation, blastocyst implantation, placental blood flow regulation, lactation, and contractile activity of the uterus" (Noor et al. 2010).

Histamine also wears a neurotransmitter hat, communicating important messages from your body to your brain. It is an excitatory neurotransmitter, which is why antihistamines can make you drowsy. Because of its excitatory effect, elevated histamine levels can contribute to anxiety, ADHD, and sleep issues.

While we definitely don't want excess histamine levels in the body, too little histamine can cause psychological and behavioral disorders. Also, with too little histamine, we will not have adequate gastric acid secretion and digestion.

Because they may not have typical allergy-like symptoms, many people do not know they have histamine issues, which are referred to as histamine intolerance. Histamine intolerance happens when histamine isn't broken down fast enough because it's coming into the body in larger quantities than the body can break down, or the body has inadequate enzyme activity to effectively clear it. When the level

DOI: 10.1201/b23201-17

of histamine in the body surpasses what it can clear, symptoms occur. Unlike food sensitivities or allergies, histamine intolerance is cumulative.

15.2 WHAT CAUSES HISTAMINE INTOLERANCE?

When investigating histamine intolerance, four main factors must be considered:

1. Histamine intake/exposure
2. Histamine production
3. Histamine receptor activity
4. The ability to clear it from the body

I like to use the analogy of a bathtub, where histamine is the water filling up the tub. Some people have diets or live in environments where it is like the faucet is on full blast constantly. This also happens when people have mast cell activation syndrome (MCAS), in which the mast cells are trigger happy and release histamine (and other mediators) at inappropriate times and in inappropriate amounts.

Some people are genetically predisposed to having smaller tubs than others. We want to make sure the drain is fully open so that the tub doesn't overflow. If it does, that is when symptoms appear. Symptomatology is determined by which side of the tub the water overflows (our four histamine receptors). Some people are genetically predisposed to having more narrow drains, and others get clogs in their drains, both of which slow down the clearance of histamine.

Let's break down the four factors.

15.3 HISTAMINE INTAKE/EXPOSURE

Histamine is found in many foods, even some of the healthiest. Aged, cured, and fermented foods are extremely high in histamine because the longer a food sits, the more histamine it will contain. These are foods like yogurt/kefir, cured deli meats, aged cheeses (including goat), sauerkraut, kombucha, vinegars (including vinegar-containing condiments like ketchup, pickles, and mayonnaise), and alcohol (especially beer and wines).

To be clear, this is *not* a blanket statement urging everyone to stay away from fermented foods. Fermented foods have numerous health benefits, especially to our microbiome, which benefit everything from immunity to cognitive functioning to fertility. However, for people with histamine intolerance, these benefits can be outweighed by the inflammation that excess histamine levels can create.

In addition to fermented food, some foods that contain high levels of histamine are:

- Nuts, especially cashews, peanuts, and walnuts
- Soured foods: sour cream, sourdough bread, and buttermilk
- Most citrus fruits
- Dried fruit
- Smoked fish

- Avocados
- Spinach
- Onions and garlic
- Tomatoes
- Eggplant

In addition to histamine-containing foods, your "tub" can get filled faster by foods, beverages, and other substances that stimulate histamine release in the body, even if they do not themselves contain high amounts of histamine. These are called histamine liberators. Foods can contain histamine and be histamine liberators at the same time.

Some foods that are histamine liberators include:

- Alcohol
- Chocolate
- Tomatoes
- Strawberries
- Nuts
- Pineapple
- Milk
- Eggs
- Fish and shellfish
- Bananas

15.4 HISTAMINE PRODUCTION

With the help of vitamin B6, mast cells convert the amino acid histidine to histamine via the enzyme histidine decarboxylase (HDC). The HDC gene is the gene that makes this enzyme, and when it is variated, it causes an upregulation in enzymatic activity. This upregulation increases the conversion of histidine to histamine, potentially causing low histidine levels and histamine levels that rise too rapidly for the body to effectively clear.

People with HDC variants who seem to have histamine intolerance might want to look at limiting high histi *dine*-containing foods rather than focusing on avoiding high histamine foods. But this requires mindful thought and interpretation of other histamine-related genes (discussed ahead) because we don't want to drive histidine too low either, as healthy levels are necessary for many functions in the body.

Histidine is critical to the growth and repair of tissue, the myelin sheath, and red blood cell production, and it protects tissue from damage from heavy metals and radiation. It also acts as an anti-inflammatory and antioxidant by inhibiting the production of proinflammatory cytokines (Wade and Tucker 1998). Histidine is critical for gastric acid secretion, and people with low histidine levels often will have hypochlorhydria, which impairs protein digestion. Because of this, it makes sense that histidine is found primarily in higher-protein foods like meat, fish, poultry, and eggs.

If you have HDC variants and symptoms of high histamine coupled with chronically low stomach acid, slow muscle repair, or cardiovascular issues (histidine is important for protecting the cardiovascular tissue), consider slowing down HDC activity, as opposed to lowering histamine levels, to spare HDC. Low-histamine diets may only deal with half the histamine puzzle.

15.5 ACTION STEPS TO COMPENSATE FOR HDC GENE UPREGULATION AND SLOW HISTIDINE-TO-HISTAMINE CONVERSION

There are some nutrients and beneficial bacteria that can help to inhibit HDC activity so we can slow conversion to effectively raise histidine to where we need it yet keep histamine levels in check.

- EGCG from green tea has been shown not only to have potent anti-inflammatory and anti-tumoral effects but also to inactivate HDC (Melgarejo et al. 2010). If someone has a need for histidine and/or a high protein diet but has HDC SNPs that push histidine into histamine too quickly, EGCG can inhibit the conversion of histidine to histamine.
- Taking quercetin, a plant pigment (flavonoid) and antioxidant, 30 minutes before a meal can help as well. Quercetin is considered one of the most potent ways to prevent the mast cells from releasing histamine (Park et al. 2008).
- I stated earlier that B6 is a cofactor for HDC. Many people are deficient in B6. If you need B6 but have HDC variants that increase the conversion of histidine to histamine, you won't want to take large doses of B6. You can compensate with naringenin. Naringenin is a citrus-derived flavonoid found in grapefruit, pomelo, and bergamot that has antiviral and anti-inflammatory properties. Naringenin is an excellent inhibitor of HDC.
- Magnesium is a cofactor for and regulates histidine decarboxylase (HDC) activity.
- We outsource a huge number of biological functions to our gut bacteria. The probiotic Bifidobacterium longum has a long list of health benefits, but its cool party trick is that it decreases expression of HDC and the HRH1 receptor (more on this ahead). To increase B. longum in the gut, we can feed it with prebiotics and fiber.

15.6 HISTAMINE RECEPTOR ACTIVITY

There are four histamine receptors and, therefore, four histamine receptor genes (HRH1, HRH2, HRH3, HRH4). When histamine is released by mast cells and gets in the presence of a histamine receptor, it can be activated. The symptoms you get from histamine depend on which histamine receptors are being activated.

Although you don't need to have any genetic polymorphisms on your histamine receptor genes to be activated, having an SNP on a histamine receptor gene will be like having that side of the tub be shorter, allowing the water to overflow that side.

15.7 MEET THE HISTAMINE RECEPTORS

Histamine receptors are widely expressed in the body, and each has specific functions.

- HRH1 receptor activation plays a role in causing vessels to vasodilate, bronchial constriction, mucus secretion, and platelet aggregation.
- HRH2 receptor activation activity takes place mainly in the gastrointestinal tract, playing a role in gastric acid secretion, nausea, and abdominal pain. It also plays a role in heart rate modulation.
- HRH3 receptor activation involves the central nervous system, affecting body temperature, learning, sleep/wake cycles, appetite, release of dopamine and norepinephrine in the brain, and memory. Symptoms can include headache, dizziness, and nausea. High H3 receptor activity has been associated with neurodegenerative diseases.
- HRH4 receptor activity has effects throughout the body. It seems to be important for mast cell activation syndrome. H4 activity involves immune response and inflammatory health conditions.

15.8 A NOTE ON ANTIHISTAMINES

Most antihistamine drugs on the market work on the H1 and H2 receptors. The important point to remember here is that these drugs don't actually reduce histamine; they only block receptor activity. This is like putting tape over a keyhole. If histamine can't bind to the receptor, there may be more free histamine wandering around in the blood, which can activate histamine receptors elsewhere. If antihistamines are used for prolonged periods of time, overall histamine levels will rise because if the body isn't getting the histamine response it wants, it will start releasing more histamine.

Remember that histamine is needed for gastric acid production. Antihistamines that are H2 blockers lower histamine in the gastrointestinal tract, which lowers gastric acid production levels, which can hinder protein digestion. We need the stomach to be very acidic to kill bacteria, viruses, mold, and parasites that hitch a ride on the food we eat. Low stomach acid can open the door for these opportunistic pathogens, as well as leading to nutrient depletion, acid reflux, malabsorption, and low neurotransmitter levels.

When we take histamine blockers, it is like tilting the tub so that the water doesn't spill out on one particular side, but it doesn't get rid of the histamine. We want to drain the histamine, not tilt the tub to keep it from overflowing. Additionally, studies have shown that people can develop dementia-type problems with long-term use of histamine blockers (Boustani et al. 2007).

I want to be clear that I am not saying not to take antihistamines. If someone finds relief with antihistamines, leave those in place while starting to do the foundational work to lower levels in the body so that the drug can be slowly tapered off.

15.9 THE ABILITY TO CLEAR HISTAMINE FROM THE BODY

If we think of histamine as the water that fills the tub and the receptors as the four sides of the tub, the ability to clear it can be thought of as one drain hole at the bottom of the tub that splits into four separate pipes that run the water out of the bathroom.

The four drainpipes are the four ways our bodies clear histamine: DAO activity, methylation, acetylation, and glucuronidation. I wrote about methylation, the phase 2 liver detoxification pathway in Chapter 4, and acetylation and glucuronidation in Chapter 13.

The first and most well-known method to clear histamine is via the enzyme diamine oxidase (DAO), made by the amiloride binding protein 1 (ABP1) gene. This gene is also referred to as the amine oxidase copper containing (AOC1) gene. Diamine oxidase was formerly called histaminase. When we have variants in the ABP1/AOC1 gene, our diamine oxidase production will be slowed.

While there are numerous ABP1 variants that one can have, having the G allele of ABP1 rs1049793 can create a high predisposition for decreased DAO production and can cause a big block in histamine clearance.

Important side note: I want to clarify a common mistake that even some of the most well-respected people in the functional genomics and histamine communities make. They state that the DAO gene is what makes diamine oxidase. This is incorrect. The DAO gene makes an enzyme called D-amino acid oxidase and is also known as the DAAO gene. The DAO gene is associated with the synthesis of dopamine and may play a role in schizophrenia (Kawazoe et al. 2007).

The diamine oxidase enzyme degrades histamine and is primarily produced in the intestinal lining, as well as the kidneys and thymus. When we are pregnant, our placentas produce a very significant amount. Diamine oxidase breaks down both endogenously produced histamine and dietary histamine.

15.10 NUTRITIONAL COFACTORS TO SUPPORT DAO ACTIVITY

The activity of DAO is also dependent on vitamin B6. There can be a delicate balance between B6 increasing HDC activity to make histamine and B6 being required to make the histamine-degrading enzyme DAO. This is where knowing your genetic profile can be very helpful in knowing what sort of protocol to implement.

Magnesium is helpful in the metabolism of histamine. Magnesium is essential for so many reactions in the body. It helps to make DAO, and in animal studies, deficiency in magnesium caused a rise in histamine. My favorite forms to supplement with are magnesium threonate, glycinate, malate, and taurate.

DAO is a copper-containing enzyme. Since copper is a required cofactor for the production of DAO, insufficient copper will cause insufficient amounts of DAO to be made. Refer to Chapter 8 to read more about copper levels in the body, copper's antagonistic relationship with zinc, and copper-related genes. For additional information on copper-related genes and their biochemical pathways, refer to Appendix 8C.

Refer to Appendix 2 for information on superoxide dismutase (SOD) and Appendix 15 for a little additional information on the relationship between SOD and histamine.

15.11 EXCESS HISTAMINE CAUSES POOR GUT HEALTH (AND VICE VERSA), WHICH CAUSES LOW DAO, WHICH CAUSES ELEVATED HISTAMINE

Low levels of DAO correlate with poor mucosal integrity. Because the microvilli in the intestinal lining secrete DAO, when we have intestinal inflammation or villous atrophy, DAO production is hindered, causing more susceptibility to histamine intolerance disorders. When this damage is coupled with less-than-optimal beneficial gut bacteria that help clear histamine, the effects are compounded. Damage to the microvilli will also affect nutrient absorption, paving the way for nutrient deficiencies. And since certain nutrients are needed for DAO production, this can be a vicious cycle.

People who have celiac and non-celiac gluten sensitivity will often have inadequate DAO production despite robust genes (no variants), so we cannot rely only on genetics to see if someone may or may not have histamine intolerance. This is why I repeatedly say that your genes are not a diagnosis and that we cannot just "treat the SNP."

Our gut barrier is made of cells that are tightly lined up next to each other. Tight junctions are the areas where two cells meet to form that barrier. Healthy tight junctions are critical for protecting the body from foreign substances. There are many factors that cause tight junctions to lose integrity, opening them (a condition called "leaky gut" or intestinal permeability) to create space for foreign substances and undigested proteins to pass into the blood. When tight junctions remain open for prolonged periods of time, they can trigger an immune response because the immune system will constantly be reacting to "foreign invaders" that keep getting into the blood. This can result in the immune system being on such high alert that it starts attacking anything that resembles the original offender, even the body's own tissue, and may ultimately lead to autoimmune diseases. Some factors that are known to compromise tight junctions include glyphosate (Samsel and Seneff 2013), poor diet, alcohol (Wang et al. 2014), many medications (including NSAIDs and antibiotics), stress, overgrowth of harmful organisms (bacteria, yeast, parasites), food sensitivities, and excess histamine.

15.12 DAO BLOCKERS

In addition to histamine-containing substances and histamine liberators, certain foods, beverages, and other substances can contribute to histamine intolerance by blocking DAO activity. These include:

- Alcohol
- Black tea
- Cocoa
- Energy drinks
- Green tea

- Maté tea
- Various pharmaceutical drugs (analgesics, antibiotics, etc.)

15.13 METHYLATION OF HISTAMINE

Another method by which histamine is cleared from the body is via methylation. I wrote all about methylation in Chapter 4.

Before histamine can be degraded by DAO, the methylation-dependent enzyme histamine N-methyltransferase (HNMT) has to inactivate it in the intracellular space of cells. The HNMT enzyme, coded for by the HNMT gene, is about as commonly discussed as diamine oxidase (DAO).

If DAO activity is compromised by suboptimal gut health or genetic polymorphisms in the ABP1/AOC1 gene, then more demand will be placed on the HNMT enzyme, potentially placing more burden on other methyltransferase genes, such as PEMT (refer to Chapter 10 and Appendix 11A) and COMT, which degrades estrogen and catecholamine neurotransmitters, in addition to histamine. Remember that estrogen and histamine have a feed-forward relationship, so if estrogen is not properly cleared, higher levels will result in elevations in histamine. The DUTCH test measures how well you are methylating your estrogen (although it does not have any markers for histamine).

S-Adenosyl-methionine (SAMe), the universal methyl donor, is the key player in methylation and a required cofactor for HNMT activity. Inflammation from free radicals inhibits SAMe production, causing fewer methyl groups to be available. SNPs in the MAT1 gene, which converts methionine into SAMe, can also hinder SAMe production, which will affect methylation and, therefore, HNMT activity.

15.14 TESTING FOR HISTAMINE INTOLERANCE

Aside from measuring the DAO enzyme levels in the blood, one commonly used way to measure histamine is via a whole blood histamine test. I have, however, seen some results that question this reliability, but whole blood histamine levels way outside the ideal range of 40 to 70 ng/mL, according to William Walsh (Walsh 2014), will likely give some clues as to what's going on.

Since histamine is degraded in part by methylation, a roundabout way to assess histamine levels is through measuring methylation ability. This can either be done by measuring homocysteine (the ideal range in functional medicine is considered to be 6 to 8 umol/L) or, more thoroughly, via a methylation plasma test, which includes homocysteine, SAMe, and methionine, among other helpful markers. If results show high homocysteine coupled with high histamine, there is likely a methylation issue that can be addressed by supporting methylation to break down histamine. If homocysteine is lower or normal and histamine is high, then DAO insufficiency due to gut issues or SNPs in the ABP1 gene is likely the culprit. However, upregulated histidine (HDC) activity should also be taken into consideration.

See Figure 15.1 for how homocysteine (HCY) is seated at an important intersection in the methylation pathway.

If histamine intolerance is a problem despite methylation status looking good, the next culprits in the histamine clearance pathway would be MAOA and MAOB

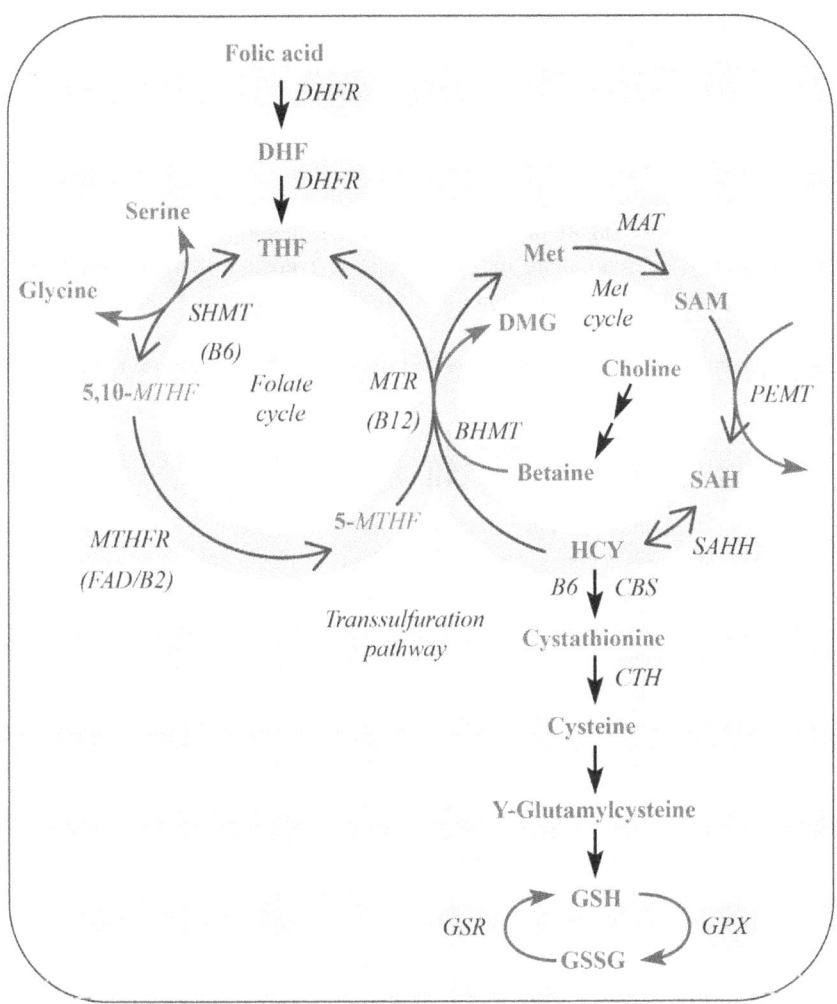

FIGURE 15.1 Homocysteine (HCY) sits at the intersection of the methionine cycle and the transsulfuration pathway. The transsulfuration pathway's ultimate job is to turn homocysteine into glutathione. The methionine cycle's primary job is to make sure homocysteine is recycled back up into SAMe, which drives methylation.

sluggishness, as they play an additional role in degrading histamine after HNMT does its thing.

MAOA and MAOB are enzymes that process amines in the body, including histamine. If someone has variants in HNMT and MAOA and/or MAOB genes, they will likely have a significant degree of impairment in histamine degradation. If these enzymes aren't functioning properly, then things can get backed up and affect the HNMT activity, resulting in elevated histamine levels. Here are a few action steps to help support HNMT activity, which can help compensate for MAOA and MAOB variants and overall histamine intolerance.

- Consider supplementing with DAO, which is usually derived from porcine kidney. This will "lighten the load" for the HNMT enzyme.
- Consider supplementing with SAMe; however, be careful not to push methyl donation too quickly, as that can backfire. This is where thoughtful interpretation of the methylation pathway genes must take place.
- Consider supporting methylation indirectly through phosphatidylcholine or creatine, which can spare methyl groups so there are more for breaking down histamine, estrogen, and other things that methylation activity helps detoxify.
- Stress can exacerbate allergies, so supporting the stress response with adaptogenic herbs can be very helpful.

15.15 ACETYLATION OF HISTAMINE

In Chapter 13 (appendix), I described the N-acetyltransferase enzymes, coded for by the NAT1 and NAT2 genes. They are involved in the metabolism of many substances that we are exposed to on a daily basis. These include xenobiotics, automobile exhaust, pesticides, caffeine, smoked/charred meats, and some medications. Histamine is also cleared through this phase 2 liver detox pathway.

The NAT genes take the acetyl group from acetyl CoA and transfer it to the toxin or chemical compound in the phase 2 liver detoxification process of acetylation. Adequate acetyl-CoA and NAT gene function is needed for proper acetylation. The NAT genes also help clear systemic mold, fungus, and/or yeast. I talk more about mold and mycotoxins in Chapter 7. Variants in the NAT genes can affect histamine clearance, and so can ACAT and PANK genetic variants.

Pantethine is the biologically active form of vitamin B5. It is made by the PANK gene and is a cofactor for NAT gene activity, so adequate levels of pantethine will help clear histamine via the acetylation pathway.

With the help of niacin (vitamin B3) as a cofactor, the ALDH2 gene also plays a role in the clearance of histamine, although it is most known for its role in processing acetaldehyde from alcohol. If there is sluggishness in the ALDH2 gene, acetaldehyde won't be efficiently broken down, and the HNMT and DAO enzymes will be called on to step in. This can take away from their primary job of degrading histamine. Refer to Chapter 13 for ways to support the acetylation pathway.

15.16 GLUCURONIDATION OF HISTAMINE

Also discussed in Chapter 13, the glucuronidation pathway is, in my opinion, the unsung hero of phase 2 liver detoxification. Most known for its significant role in clearing estrogen and mycotoxins, it is also responsible for the clearance of histamine.

The UGT1A4 gene is a major player in the clearance of amines, including tyramine, dopamine, and histamine. Refer to Chapter 13 for ways to support the glucuronidation pathway.

As you can now see, there are multiple ways that histamine is cleared by the body. It seems to be that the more important it is for something to be within specific ranges in the body, the more backup pathways, or "checks and balances," our bodies have to ensure that happens.

15.17 PROBIOTICS: HARMFUL AND HELPFUL

A well-balanced microbiome will ensure proper histamine degradation. However, not all probiotics will be beneficial for someone dealing with histamine intolerance. While some strains of probiotics help degrade histamine, others are actually histamine producing. A few histamine-producing strains are *Lactobacillus casei*, *Lactobacillus reuteri* (Mu et al. 2018), and *Lactobacillus bulgaricus* (Deepika Priyadarshani and Rakshit 2011), also called L. delbrueckii subsp. bulgaricus (TISTR 895). These strains are commonly found in most yogurts and fermented food, along with the *Leuconostoc mesenteroides* and *Pediococcus pentosaceus* strains.

Some strains known to help degrade histamine are *Bifidobacterium infantis*, *Lactobacillus rhamnosus*, *Lactobacillus plantarum*, and *Bifidobacterium longum*.

It will be good to keep these strains in mind next time you purchase probiotics; however, there are a few probiotic supplements on the market that are marketed specifically for supporting histamine degradation, so you know those will likely be a safe bet.

15.18 HISTAMINE AND REPRODUCTIVE OUTCOMES

I have mentioned a few times in this book that histamine and estrogen have a direct relationship, in which elevations in one cause a rise in the other. Concurrently, elevated estrogen may downregulate DAO activity (Fogel 1986). This is why some women experience histamine intolerance symptoms (headache/migraine, vomiting, diarrhea, etc.) right around ovulation and again about a week before menstruation when estrogen levels are at their highest. See Figure 15.2. In fact, there are studies that demonstrate relationships between histamine and endometriosis (Binda et al. 2017). Endometriosis, a manifestation of estrogen dominance, is an inflammatory condition that activates mast cells to release histamine. Interestingly, progesterone has been shown in studies to inhibit the release of histamine (Muñoz-Cruz et al. 2015). I am not saying that histamine is bad; it is only problematic in excess. Studies in rodents suggest that histamine plays important roles in normal ovulation, blastocyst implantation, and the contractile activity of the uterus (Szelag et al. 2002).

Histamine plays a much larger part in reproduction than I ever could have given thought to! As important as I have found histamine/DAO balance to be for implantation and pregnancy, the connection is unfortunately not often discussed, despite there being numerous studies on the topic.

Menstrual cycle

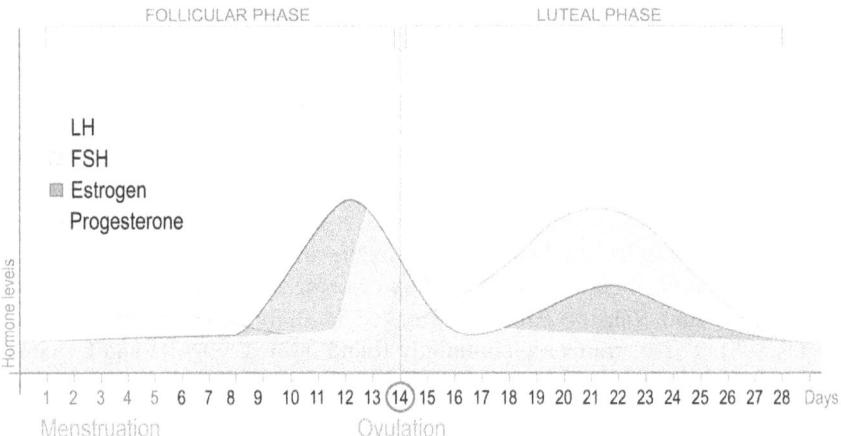

FIGURE 15.2 The menstrual cycle: Estrogen is at its highest levels right before ovulation and again about a week before menstruation begins.

The histamine/DAO balance is critical for successful conception and uncomplicated pregnancy. This delicate balance is thought to take place to protect both the pregnant woman and her fetus from excessive amounts of histamine (Carrington et al. 1972).

It is thought that histamine may play an important role in implantation, allowing the embryo to invade the uterine lining. Histamine is also important for placenta development (Woidacki et al. 2014). Total blood histamine levels are highest during the earlier parts of the first trimester and begin to lower as DAO levels begin to increase. DAO activity peaks somewhere between 12 and 24 weeks of gestation (Maintz et al. 2008).

The placenta produces a high concentration of DAO. Levels can become 500 times those of non-pregnant women (Maintz and Novak 2007). It is thought that the placenta produces amounts this high to keep histamine from entering maternal or fetal circulation (Noor et al. 2010).

Plenty of studies reflect elevations in histamine and/or inadequate levels of DAO being linked to miscarriage, preterm labor, preterm delivery, preeclampsia, intrauterine growth retardation (IUGR) (Szukiewicz et al. 1999), and hyperemesis gravidarum.

I had a client, "Cindy," come to me after having six miscarriages. When she came to me, her periods were all over the place, and so was her mood. I recommended genetic testing early on in our visits together. While we waited for her results to come in, we worked on getting her periods to be healthy, regular, and uneventful by addressing blood sugar, cutting back on her weekly jogging distance, and cleaning up her diet and personal care products. She didn't have any obvious symptoms of histamine intolerance, like seasonal allergies or allergic reactions, but her genetics showed a good number of variants in the HNMT and ABP1 genes. Although everything seemed to be normal and healthy, histamine was the "hidden rock" we needed to explore as a cause for her repeated miscarriages. Along with a lower histamine diet, we slowly started supporting the HNMT with a bioavailable vitamin B complex and added in a DAO enzyme supplement. This did the trick, and she finally made it past the first trimester and went on to have a healthy baby!

As you can see, histamine can be a very revealing aspect to investigate if someone is having issues with conceiving or sustaining a healthy pregnancy. Histamine ties into hormonal balance, DAO balance, placental health and activity, and successful pregnancies.

There are other ways to support histamine intolerance besides cutting out all moderately high-- and high-histamine-containing foods forever. There are many different plant compounds that are known mast cell stabilizers and natural antihistamines. Here are just a few.

ACTION STEPS

- Experiment with a low-histamine diet for about two to four weeks. Due to the elimination of some very nutritious foods, I would not recommend a long-term low-histamine diet unless you've spoken with a knowledgeable practitioner about the pros and cons.
- Supplement with diamine oxidase enzyme (DAO). This supplement should be taken with meals to help degrade the histamine the food may contain. Supplemental DAO is made from porcine kidney protein extract, so if you have any allergy to pork, you should not take DAO.
- Flavonoids like luteolin, quercetin, and rutin are known to help with histamine intolerance. Some practitioners recommend taking quercetin and other mast cell stabilizers 30 minutes before each meal and at bedtime.
- Bromelain is an inflammation-lowering enzyme that is derived from pineapple core.
- Stinging nettles leaf blocks histamine production (Kregiel et al. 2018) and works similarly to over-the-counter antihistamines that block histamine receptor activity.
- Support methylation, glucuronidation, and acetylation pathways.
- Work on improving the health of the gut – both the structural integrity of the gut lining and the microflora that reside in the gut.
- It would be good to get a baseline of histamine/DAO activity before pregnancy and again at around six weeks gestation if histamine is thought to be a culprit in reproductive challenges.

REFERENCES

Binda, Maria Mercedes, Jacques Donnez, and Marie-Madeleine Dolmans. 2017. "Targeting mast cells: a new way to treat endometriosis." *Expert Opinion on Therapeutic Targets* 21, no. 1, 67–75.

Boustani, Malaz, Kathleen S. Hall, Kathleen A. Lane, Hisham Aljadhey, Sujuan Gao, Frederick Unverzagt, Michael D. Murray, Adesola Ogunniyi, and Hugh Hendrie. 2007. "The association between cognition and histamine-2 receptor antagonists in African Americans." *Journal of the American Geriatrics Society* 55, no. 8, 1248–1253.

Carrington, Elsie R., Gertrude J. Frishmuth, M. Jane Oesterling, Fae M. Adams, and Susan E. Cox. 1972. "Gestational and postpartum plasma diamine oxidase values." *Obstetrics & Gynecology* 39, no. 3, 426–430.

Deepika Priyadarshani, Wadu Mesthri, and Sudip K. Rakshit. 2011. "Screening selected strains of probiotic lactic acid bacteria for their ability to produce biogenic amines (histamine and tyramine)." *International Journal of Food Science & Technology* 46, no. 10, 2062–2069.

Fogel, W. A. 1986. "Diamine oxidase (DAO) and female sex hormones." *Agents and Actions* 18, no. 1, 44–45.

Kawazoe, Tomoya, Hwan Ki Park, Sanae Iwana, Hideaki Tsuge, and Kiyoshi Fukui. 2007. "Human D-amino acid oxidase: an update and review." *The Chemical Record* 7, no. 5, 305–315.

Kregiel, Dorota, Ewelina Pawlikowska, and Hubert Antolak. 2018. "Urtica spp.: ordinary plants with extraordinary properties." *Molecules* 23, no. 7, 1664.

Maintz, Laura, and Natalija Novak. 2007. "Histamine and histamine intolerance." *The American Journal of Clinical Nutrition* 85, no. 5, 1185–1196.

Maintz, Laura, Verena Schwarzer, Thomas Bieber, Katrin van der Ven, and Natalija Novak. 2008. "Effects of histamine and diamine oxidase activities on pregnancy: a critical review." *Human Reproduction Update* 14, no. 5, 485–495.

Melgarejo, Esther, Miguel Ángel Medina, Francisca Sánchez-Jiménez, and José Luis Urdiales. 2010. "Targeting of histamine producing cells by EGCG: a green dart against inflammation?" *Journal of Physiology and Biochemistry* 66, no. 3, 265–270.

Mu, Qinghui, Vincent J. Tavella, and Xin M. Luo. 2018. "Role of Lactobacillus reuteri in human health and diseases." *Frontiers in Microbiology* 9, 757.

Muñoz-Cruz, Samira, Yolanda Mendoza-Rodríguez, Karen E. Nava-Castro, Lilián Yepez-Mulia, and Jorge Morales-Montor. 2015. "Gender-related effects of sex steroids on histamine release and FcεRI expression in rat peritoneal mast cells." *Journal of Immunology Research* 2015.

Noor, Nasreen, Trivendra Tripathi, Shagufta Moin, and Abdul Faiz Faizy. 2010. "Possible effect of histamine in physiology of female reproductive function: An updated review." *Biomedical Aspects of Histamine* 395–405.

Park, Hyo-Hyun, Soyoung Lee, Hee-Young Son, Seung-Bin Park, Mi-Sun Kim, Eun-Ju Choi, Thoudam S. K. Singh, et al. 2008. "Flavonoids inhibit histamine release and expression of proinflammatory cytokines in mast cells." *Archives of Pharmacal Research* 31, no. 10, 1303–1311.

Samsel, Anthony, and Stephanie Seneff. 2013. "Glyphosate, pathways to modern diseases II: Celiac sprue and gluten intolerance." *Interdisciplinary Toxicology* 6, no. 4, 159–184.

Szelag, Adam, Anna Merwid-Lad, and Małgorzata Trocha. 2002. "Histamine receptors in the female reproductive system. Part I. Role of the mast cells and histamine in female reproductive system." *Ginekologia Polska* 73, no. 7, 627–635.

Szukiewicz, D., A. Szukiewicz, D. Maslinska, P. Poppe, M. Gujski, and M. Olszewski. 1999. "Mast cells and histamine in intrauterine growth retardation-relation to the development of placental microvessels." *Inflammation Research* 48, no. 13, 41–42.

Wade, A. Michael, and Hugh N. Tucker. 1998. "Antioxidant characteristics of L-histidine." *The Journal of Nutritional Biochemistry* 9, no. 6, 308–315.

Walsh, William J. 2014. *Nutrient Power: Heal Your Biochemistry and Heal your Brain.* Simon and Schuster.

Wang, Ying, Jing Tong, Bing Chang, Baifang Wang, Dai Zhang, and Bingyuan Wang. 2014. "Effects of alcohol on intestinal epithelial barrier permeability and expression of tight junction-associated proteins." *Molecular Medicine Reports* 9, no. 6, 2352–2356.

Woidacki, Katja, Ana Claudia Zenclussen, and Frank Siebenhaar. 2014. "Mast cell-mediated and associated disorders in pregnancy: a risky game with an uncertain outcome?" *Frontiers in Immunology* 5, 231.

16 Additional Support

Tighten Up Your Blood Sugar Levels: Why Addressing All the Previous Steps Will Help Balance Blood Sugar

I want to start this chapter by stating that addressing all the steps from previous weeks will help balance blood sugar. Blood sugar balance is easily dysregulated by inflammation and stressors of all sorts. The reason I made this topic "Additional Support" is that doing the action steps in previous weeks should have moved the needle for regulating blood sugar. Some people still need support even after implementing the previous action steps. This chapter can help.

16.1 BLOOD SUGAR IMBALANCE = RISE IN CORTISOL = REPRODUCTIVE PROBLEMS

The ability of the body to properly deal with blood sugar is integral for wellness and fertility. So many reproductive issues have roots in blood sugar dysregulation (technically called dysglycemia). Dysregulations in blood sugar typically are from hypoglycemia or insulin resistance, both of which can lead to metabolic syndrome or, ultimately, type 2 diabetes. One out of every five Americans has metabolic syndrome, which is associated with higher risks of gestational diabetes, high blood pressure, preeclampsia, and preterm labor (Marsh and Hecker 2014).

The reason reproductive issues are rooted in problems with blood sugar regulation is because cortisol, insulin, and our sex hormones are all intimately connected.

Our bodies still react to a stressor in the same way they always have since humanity began. When the body senses danger, cortisol acts to prepare the body for a fight-or-flight response by flooding it with glucose, eliciting a rise in blood sugar. This glucose prepares to give the cells the required fuel they need, especially in large muscles like the legs and heart, so we can either run away from or fight the source of danger.

The pancreas produces insulin in response to elevated blood sugar to shuttle the sugar from the blood into the cells to be used for energy. If, as in the standard American diet, either too much sugar is consumed in a short period of time causing an excessive release of insulin (venti caramel latte, anyone?), or the pancreas is having to secrete insulin too often. This can cause insulin receptors ("keyholes" on the cell that insulin fits into) to get inflamed and shut down (insulin resistance), so cells start to starve for nutrition/energy since the sugar isn't getting in. This can lead to some gnarly cravings,

DOI: 10.1201/b23201-18

by the way. Insulin – too much and/or too often – elicits a cortisol response, and this cycle keeps cortisol levels consistently elevated, leading to chronic inflammation.

The pancreas will keep signaling for insulin to be secreted, but because of the insulin resistant receptors, the sugar ends up staying in the blood and getting stored as fat or glycogen in the liver, potentially leading to non-alcoholic fatty liver disease (NAFLD); there is a definite connection between NAFLD and diabetes. The excess fat causes estrogen to be produced, which throws the estrogen/progesterone ratio off, leading to estrogen dominance and tossing the dice for all the wonky period and reproductive issues a woman would never want.

Symptoms of insulin resistance:

- Inability to lose weight
- Cravings for sugar
- Fatigue especially after meals
- Constant hunger
- Mid-afternoon slump
- Migrating aches and pains
- Upper abdominal obesity
- Increased fat storage
- High cholesterol and triglycerides
- Low thyroid
- Estrogen dominance
- PCOS (accompanied by acne, facial hair, infertility)

Similarly, when the blood sugar gets too low (hypoglycemia), the adrenal glands go into emergency mode because they start to panic about where their energy will come from, and cortisol is called on.

Fit people with no obvious symptoms of blood sugar issues (typical symptoms are fat accumulation around waist, getting "hangry," high fasting glucose) can absolutely have blood sugar dysregulation. When I was a bike messenger boozehound in my 20s, sometimes when I was ovulating, it felt like a broomstick was being jabbed into my left ovary every time I went to sit down. Alcohol metabolizes into sugar, and I was having numerous beers each night. Even though I was in incredible shape, didn't eat much sugar, and had no other signs of blood sugar issues, this was a huge flag.

There are numerous ways to optimize your blood sugar functioning. Aside from symptoms that can be very clear in telling you if you have blood sugar/insulin issues, there are a few tests you can request from your practitioner. Many folks have gotten fasting glucose checked at some point in life, but the "normal" range is broad. I prefer to see numbers between 80 and 90 for optimal functioning, which is better than "normal." Also, fasting insulin should, ideally, be below 5 or 6.

16.2 THE BLOOD SUGAR ROLLER COASTER CONSTANTLY RELIES ON CORTISOL TO SAVE THE DAY

Inflammation goes hand in hand with elevated cortisol. I've mentioned that inflammation can be caused from just about anything that causes imbalance in the body, like high blood sugar, elevated insulin, toxins, fungal overgrowth, pathogens, and oxidative stress. Basically, what this whole book has discussed so far.

In the same way that cells can become resistant to the hormone insulin in the presence of inflammation, inflammation also can cause other types of hormone resistance. This happens when hormones are being produced just fine, but the cellular receptors are not hearing the hormones knocking at the door to come in, so the end result is the same as not producing enough. However, the flip side of that is that the levels of the hormones being produced can become too high.

Dysglycemia and insulin resistance can stimulate androgen production in the ovaries, increasing testosterone levels. Aromatase is an enzyme that converts testosterone to estrogen. Too much aromatase activity causes estrogen dominance and the issues that it comes with, like fibroids and endometriosis. Aromatase is upregulated by inflammation. In women with endometriosis, the extrauterine endometrial tissue increases aromatase, compounding the problem.

Certain pesticides are known to upregulate aromatase activity as well (Bretveld et al. 2006).

Insulin resistance is one of many causes of inflammation and aromatase activity, and it also causes storage of fat. Fat produces estrogen. If we fix the insulin resistance, we can often fix the estrogen problem (Figure 16.1).

It is widely known that PCOS is one of the most common causes of infertility (Services 2019) and increases the risk of miscarriage and pregnancy complications (National Institute of Child Health and Human Development n.d.). It is not as well known that PCOS is very related to metabolic issues like insulin resistance and glucose intolerance and subsequent metabolic syndrome. In the US, almost 50% of women with PCOS present with metabolic syndrome (Carmina et al. 2006). When a woman has elevated insulin, it not only raises cortisol, but it also causes an enzyme called 17,20-lyase to increase testosterone production, which can lead to polycystic ovary syndrome (PCOS).

In addition to impaired fertility, PCOS also causes women to grow hair where they don't want it and to lose it where they do want it. This is due to increased testosterone, as well as inflammation from poor blood sugar regulation (or numerous other sources of inflammation).

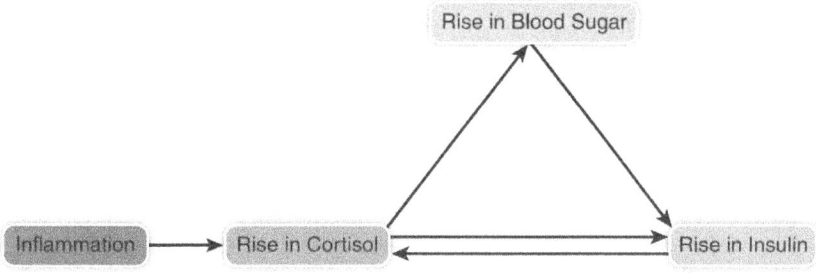

FIGURE 16.1 Inflammation fuels blood sugar dysregulation. Keeping your blood sugar and insulin sensitivity in check can help keep estrogen from dominating you.

To add to the hormonal imbalance, if the cells aren't getting the fuel they need, the downstream effect is that all the glands that produce our hormones don't get the nourishment they need to work, ultimately compounding the hormonal disharmony.

So balancing blood sugar to keep cortisol from being called on is something we have control over and can be the first step in getting hormones into balance.

ACTION STEPS

Here are some actionable tips for getting blood sugar balance under control.

- Diet, of course, is foundational. As everyone already knows, bad fats and refined flours and grains contribute to poor health effects and wonky blood sugar. High sugar and carbs stress the adrenals, as I just talked about.
- If your blood sugar balance is easily upset, pair fat and/or protein with your carbohydrates. Focus more on fat- and protein-based breakfasts.
- Know the amount of carbs your body can handle for a healthy blood sugar response.
- Sleep good amounts. I am someone who needs my sleep, and my ability to handle stress greatly depends on getting enough sleep.
- Exercise regularly, even if it's only for a few minutes each day; that's better than none. Do not exercise to the point that you feel tired or irritable a couple hours afterwards. This type of exercise stresses your adrenals.
- B vitamins are needed to convert glucose into ATP. ATP is essential in strengthening and protecting our eggs.
  - Some folks might consider vitamin B6 – in its activated form, pyridoxal-5-phosphate (P5P) – to be a panacea for PMS, PCOS, and even PMDD. P5P is essential for the synthesis of steroid hormones, especially progesterone (a.k.a. "pro-gestation"). It supports calming neurotransmitter production, as it is necessary for converting glutamate (excitatory neurotransmitter) into GABA (a calming neurotransmitter), and it is needed for serotonin production. B6 regulates anti-inflammatory prostaglandins and estrogen detoxification. Additionally, B6 is a cofactor for histamine metabolism. I also mentioned earlier that it is an important component of the folate cycle (as are other Bs) and also helps with oxalate metabolism.
    - The CDC found vitamin B6 to be the number one deficiency in the United States.
  - Inositol, also referred to as vitamin B8, helps keep insulin receptors working optimally so the body remains sensitive to insulin.
- Chromium is an essential trace mineral. It comes in various forms and has been shown to have a beneficial role in the regulation of insulin by enhancing its activity, as well as affecting carbohydrate, protein, and lipid metabolism. It helps metabolize sugar by shuttling it into the cell so the cell can use it to make energy. Studies have shown that type 2 diabetes is related to low blood levels of chromium and that insulin resistance usually is present with PCOS and gestational diabetes. Chromium supplementation can enhance insulin activity, improve glucose metabolism, and lower cardiovascular

disease risk, particularly in overweight individuals (Havel 2004). It can even be beneficial for sugar cravings! I prefer the polynicotinate form, also called GTF chromium (glucose tolerance factor), which has been shown to be safe and effective.

- Shatavari root. Meaning "one with 100 husbands," this herb is widely known as a female tonic that supports the reproductive system in an abundance of ways. It is considered the "Queen of Herbs" in Ayurveda due to its impressively long list of potentially beneficial properties (Alok et al. 2013). It is an adaptogenic herb that alleviates adrenal stress, sparing reproductive hormones. It is also recognized as an antioxidant (Wiboonpun et al. 2004) that helps combat oxidative stress.
- Alpha lipoic acid is an antioxidant that helps sugar convert to energy. Studies have shown it to be beneficial for fasting blood glucose levels and insulin resistance. ALA also has demonstrated positive effects on egg maturation, embryo development, and reproductive outcomes.

REFERENCES

Alok, Shashi, Sanjay Kumar Jain, Amita Verma, Mayank Kumar, Alok Mahor, and Monika Sabharwal. 2013. "Plant profile, phytochemistry and pharmacology of Asparagus racemosus (Shatavari): a review." *Asian Pacific Journal of Tropical Disease* 3, no. 3, 242–251.

Bretveld, Reini W., Chris MG Thomas, Paul TJ Scheepers, Gerhard A. Zielhuis, and Nel Roeleveld. 2006. "Pesticide exposure: the hormonal function of the female reproductive system disrupted?" *Reproductive Biology and Endocrinology* 4, no. 1, 1–14.

Carmina, Enrico, Nicola Napoli, R. A. Longo, G. B. Rini, and R. A. Lobo. 2006. "Metabolic syndrome in polycystic ovary syndrome (PCOS): lower prevalence in southern Italy than in the USA and the influence of criteria for the diagnosis of PCOS." *European Journal of Endocrinology* 154, no. 1, 141–145.

Havel, Peter J. 2004. "A scientific review: the role of chromium in insulin resistance." *Diabetes Educator* 30, no. 3, 1–14.

Marsh, Courtney A., and Erin Hecker. 2014. "Maternal obesity and adverse reproductive outcomes: reducing the risk." *Obstetrical & Gynecological Survey* 69, no. 10, 622–628.

National Institute of Child Health and Human Development. n.d. Does PCOS affect pregnancy? www.nichd.nih.gov/health/topics/pcos/more_information/FAQs/pregnancy.

US Department of Health & Human Services. 2019. Office on women's health. www.womenshealth.gov/a-z-topics/polycystic-ovary-syndrome.

Wiboonpun, Nathathai, Preecha Phuwapraisirisan, and Santi Tip-pyang. 2004. "Identification of antioxidant compound from Asparagus racemosus." *Phytotherapy Research: An International Journal Devoted to Pharmacological and Toxicological Evaluation of Natural Product Derivatives* 18, no. 9, 771–773.

17 Summing It Up/ Conclusion

Now that you have an understanding of what functional nutrigenomics is, you know that what may be nourishing and beneficial to one body can cause inflammation in another. It shines a light on why one diet or specific supplement worked wonders for someone but made someone else sick. Some incredibly beneficial foods like green smoothies and spinach can really derail someone's health while they can bring another person back from the hell of chronic disease.

Also, some diets like keto, vegan, and paleo have worked wonders for some folks while creating more problems from the get-go for others.

This is where functional genomic nutrition really proves itself. As I detailed earlier in the book, knowing what metabolic steps need to be supported (proper fat utilization, good NADPH levels, etc.) before, for example, implementing a keto diet can save someone a boatload of inflammation and puzzlement as to why the diet didn't work for them.

Additionally, in the case of whether or not you have MTHFR or other variants in the methylation cycle, you can know which forms are preferred for vitamin and mineral supplementation, as well as the right time to begin implementing them, rather than supplementing blindly and having it backfire, causing inflammation, anxiety, and/or irritation.

Addressing adrenal and limbic/HPA axis issues, inflammation, and the body's toxic load are imperative for anyone planning or trying to conceive. As you've read and now know, there are an incredible number of things that cause issues in these foundational pillars.

If the adrenals are weak or dysregulated, DHEA and pregnenolone (the precursors to sex and stress hormones) production will be inadequate. Yes, they are produced elsewhere in the body, but the adrenal glands are the primary source of production. Adrenal issues are upstream of thyroid issues, and many women may experience things like miscarriage or postpartum depression because of dysregulated adrenals and the resulting thyroid imbalance.

In this book, you've learned that many of us have genetic predispositions for weakness in detoxification pathways, and that does not bode well for the number of negative environmental factors our bodies are overwhelmed with. If our bodies are not detoxifying the scary amounts of toxins we are bombarded with each day, we will be toxic and inflamed and likely anxious and depressed, too.

While inflammation is a normal and important part of healing and response to injury and disease, too many factors are making it chronic and progressively worse in our bodies.

DOI: 10.1201/b23201-19

Paper after paper in the National Library of Medicine shows that consumer products and chemicals play a much larger part in miscarriage, infertility, and birth defects than previously believed. This only adds insult to injury when someone has been exposed to mold or has any of the root causes of inflammation that this book has detailed. Various factors such as genetic inheritance, environmental factors, and age can result in dramatic differences in how well toxic metabolites are eliminated from the body. Based on what was shared in this book, we now know that we cannot change the genes we've been given, but we can help promote the healthy expression of those genes in our offspring by living a lifestyle that does not promote inflammation and body burden.

Thinking about all the toxins and stressors we are exposed to can be absolutely and completely overwhelming. I want to say again that we are striving for improvement and progress, not perfection. Every purchase we make is a vote for the world we want to bring children into. There are always a couple more things we can improve on to bring down the total body burden. There is an app called DetoxMe that can be helpful and makes implementing non-toxic habits almost like a game!

If the cells in our body think that there is a cause for alarm or not enough energy to create a baby, they will significantly impair reproductive capacities. If the body constantly needs cortisol, it will not give the green light to bringing a child into a stressful environment. We need to squelch inflammation, make sure our bodies are energy-generating machines, and calm our limbic systems to ensure our autonomic nervous system is balanced so we can rest, digest, detox, repair, and reproduce.

Appendix 1

APPENDIX 1A: DESCRIBING THE PYRAMID FUNCTION

My favorite way to view personalized genetic information is through a cloud-based software that uses a customized functional genomic nutrition (FGN) pyramid. The bottom of the pyramid contains the foundational blocks that cover many of the things that contribute to inflammation and oxidative stress, which I detail at great length in this book, like genes related to gut health and function, histamine intolerance, iron dysregulation, and glutamate excess. The blocks in the FGN pyramid display predispositions for antioxidant production, cellular health, liver detox ability, fat utilization, and metabolism of various nutrients. To literally top it off is MTHFR, folate, and methylation, and I'll explain why this is often one of the last pieces that should be addressed (Figure 1 Appendix 1).

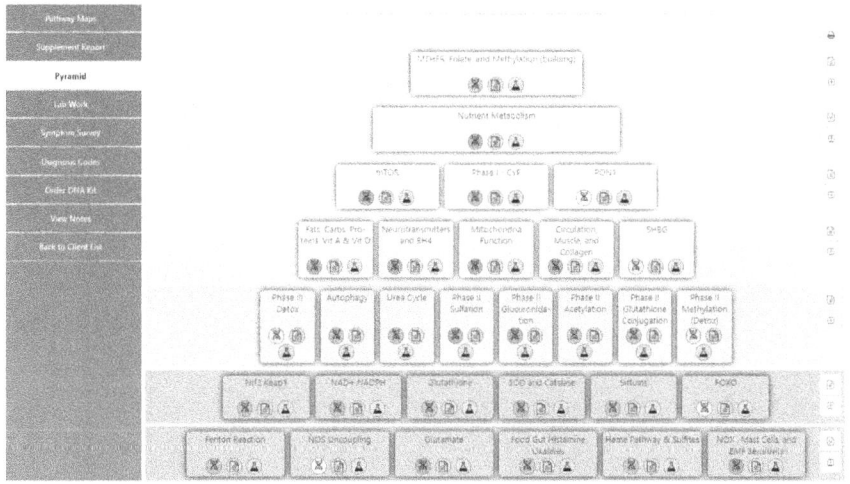

FIGURE 1 APPENDIX 1   The Functional Genomic Analysis software pyramid.

Source: Reprinted with permission from NutriGenetic Research Institute

Appendix 2

APPENDIX 2A: THE SCIENTIFIC EXPLANATION OF OXIDATIVE STRESS AND ANTIOXIDANTS

When an oxygen atom loses an electron (and its negative charge), it becomes an unstable free radical. Because electrons need to be in pairs, it will then quickly try to gain stability by stealing an electron from the nearest molecule. When the "attacked" molecule loses its electron, it becomes a free radical itself and steals an electron from another nearby molecule, beginning an extremely rapid chain reaction. Antioxidants are substances that donate electrons to stop this lightning-fast domino effect.

While we get many antioxidants from fruits and vegetables, our bodies also produce them. The top three, which I discuss in this book, are glutathione, superoxide dismutase (SOD), and catalase.

Glutathione is dubbed "the master antioxidant" because it is able to recycle itself and other antioxidants. Once an antioxidant donates an electron, its job is done, and the case is closed. This is not the case with glutathione. Glutathione can recycle itself (through a series of genetic enzymatic reactions and nutrients), and other antioxidants like vitamin C and vitamin E. There is a lot involved with glutathione production, utilization, and recycling as an antioxidant, which I discuss in Chapter 11 on antioxidants. The bonus here is that glutathione conjugation is also one of our phase 2 liver detoxification pathways (detailed in Chapter 13).

Superoxide dismutase (SOD) is one of the most abundant proteins in the body (out of thousands of proteins), punctuating its importance as a front-line protection against reactive oxygen species (ROS), which are a type of free radical. Superoxide dismutase (SOD) is an antioxidant enzyme that neutralizes the free radical superoxide ($O2-$), turning it into oxygen and hydrogen peroxide. Essentially, SOD and glutathione work like "two hands clapping": a one-two antioxidant punch.

Catalase is an antioxidant enzyme (made by the CAT gene) that further converts hydrogen peroxide (with the help of glutathione) to water and oxygen, which are essential for life (Figure 1 Appendix 2).

Free Radical   Antioxidant

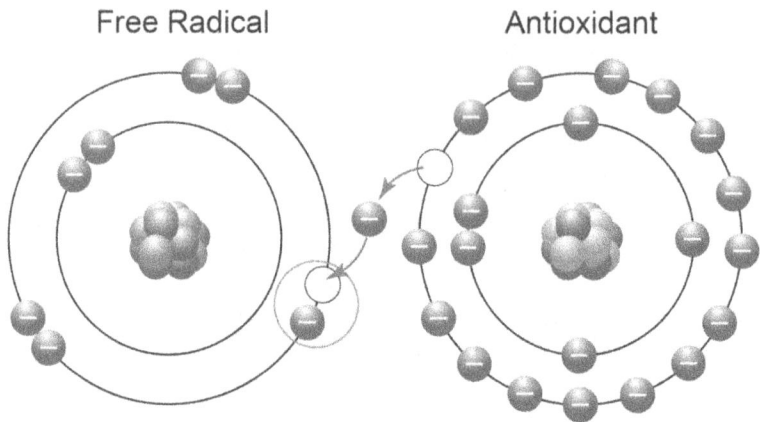

FIGURE 1 APPENDIX 2   Electrons are stable in pairs. Antioxidants donate electrons to reactive unpaired electrons.

APPENDIX 2B

Through the interpretation of urine organic acid test (OAT) results with a trained practitioner, you can get an idea of the oxidative stress load your body may be experiencing. For example, if your fats are not being properly used, they will oxidize (lipid peroxidation), causing oxidative stress, and they won't turn into hormones. If your mitochondrial markers are elevated, your mitochondria may not be efficiently making ATP, resulting in oxidative stress and low energy. Also, if glutathione levels are not adequate, that is a sign of oxidative stress. There are quite a few other markers and tests that can be a direct measurement of oxidative stress levels in the body, and they can be checked via cell, blood, saliva, and/or urine. A couple of the more common ways to assess oxidative stress load include measuring the ratio of reduced and oxidized glutathione and measuring oxidized LDL. My preferred way to measure is via 8-hydroxydeoxyguanosine (8-OHDG), a urinary measurement of oxidative stress. The DUTCH Complete test (which stands for dried urine test for comprehensive hormones) includes this marker. I mention the various benefits of the DUTCH (my favorite hormone test) in some of the pages in the main text and in Appendix 11.

Appendix 4

APPENDIX 4A

Chromosomes carry all the genetic coding for all the proteins in every cell.

Inside the nucleus of every cell are chromosomes. Chromosomes consist of genes that make up our DNA (Figure 1 Appendix 4A).

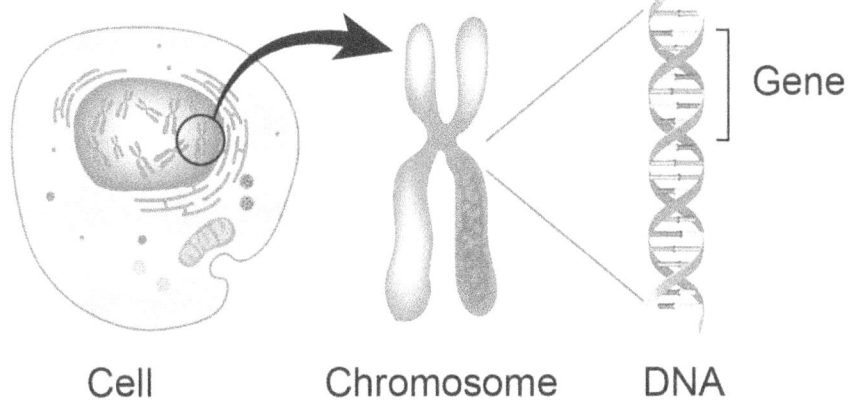

Cell   **Chromosome**   **DNA**

FIGURE 1 APPENDIX 4A   The nucleus of the cell houses the chromosomes, which are composed of DNA. Genes are short segments within a DNA strand that hold the instructions for making a protein.

DNA STRUCTURE

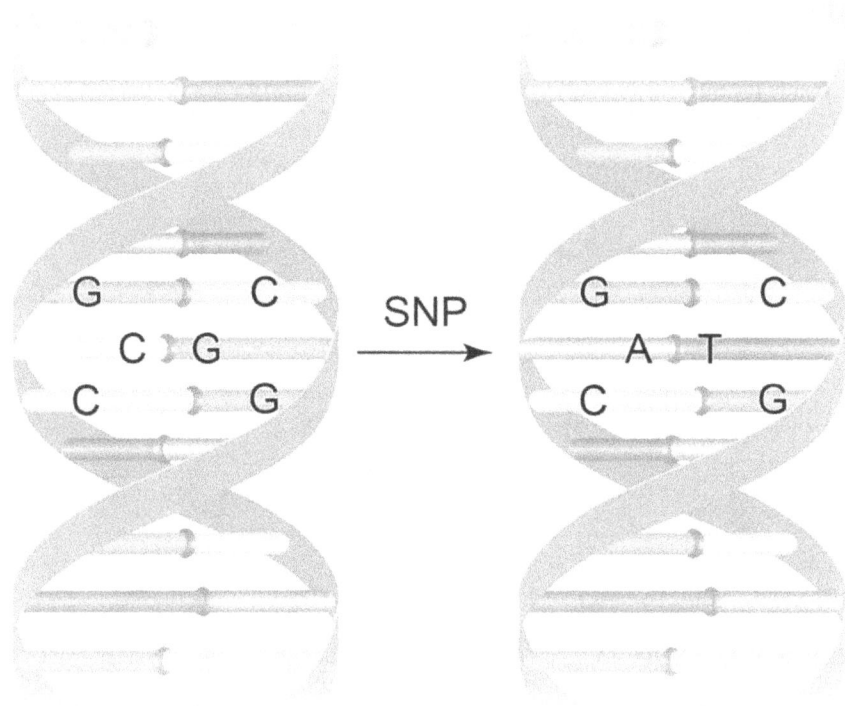

Figure 2 Appendix 4A   DNA consists of a string of four nucleotide bases: adenine, gua-nine, thymine, and cytosine (A, G, T and C) that are linked together in a double helix. Bases on opposite strands are always matched A-T and C-G. Three base pairs code for an amino acid. Single nucleotide polymorphisms, commonly referred to as SNPs (pro-nounced "snips"), are variations in a base pair of the same gene.

ANCESTRAL/WILD TYPE VERSUS RISK ALLELE

When people say that they "have the gene for [insert condition]" what they mean is that they have the SNP that predisposes them to that condition. For example, every-one has the MTHFR C677 gene, but most people have the "ancestral allele," also called the wild type allele, which is the form of the gene that has been passed down for generations. Having the "risk allele" means you have the less common variated version that's been associated with infertility, miscarriage, cardiovascular imbal-ances, and other such things. But again, just because you have the "bad" SNP doesn't mean it's doomed to express. This is where knowing your genetics *and* the influence of epigenetics can be to your advantage; you can be proactive with this knowledge.

UPREGULATION AND DOWNREGULATION, ALSO REFERRED TO AS GAIN OF FUNCTION AND LOSS OF FUNCTION

Enzymes take substance A and turn it into substance B. If there is a polymorphism, it can cause the enzyme to be produced more slowly or more rapidly. This can affect how quickly or slowly things like hormones, neurotransmitters, and drugs will be produced, utilized, and/or metabolized. MTHFR, for example, is a downregulation: i.e., it causes loss of function. If someone has a heterozygous variant (a "risk" copy from one parent), enzymatic activity may be slowed down by a certain percentage (some say about 30–40%). If a homozygous is present (a "risk" copy from both parents), this can slow down the enzymatic activity by up to 70%.

Fun fact: It's more than just the DNA blueprint that gets passed down to future generations. Research shows robust evidence that not only is the DNA inherited but the epigenetic instructions that contribute to regulating gene expression in the offspring are also inherited (Max-Planck-Gesellschaft 2017). And it's not just passed on to the next generation; scientists have observed epigenetic memories being passed down for 14 generations! (Klosin et al. 2017).

Note to practitioners: Treating SNPs is not and should not be the aim. Knowing someone's genetic code, in addition to an extraordinarily detailed case history/intake, can help you better understand some of the complexities of a case and guide your recommendations, together with their genetic potential and requirements.

There are copious amounts of other genes/enzymes in a pathway that can balance out a SNP, just as they can compound. By this, I mean that having one SNP could decrease production or transport of a substance, but another could decrease metabolism, so they may balance each other out. On the other end of the spectrum, someone could have an SNP that decreases production or transport but also have an SNP that upregulates metabolism, therefore potentially causing a huge shortage of that substance.

This is a little-known fact and it is my mission to communicate it to the world. There is now a clearer understanding of why there is so much more involved than just the MTHFR gene and even the methylation pathway. We need to look at entire pathways and how they intersect with other pathways.

Based on case history, symptoms, labs, and genetics, functional genomics looks at the functional approach: "How is the terrain off in the body?"

The objective of functional (nutri)genomics is to give the body the resources it needs to create and maintain the ideal biological environment to optimize gene expression. While traditional genetics often looks for potential disease states, functional genomics looks for potential impairment of function and helps find the best nutritional intervention to support balance of function. Remember when I said enzymes require nutritional cofactors? This is how we get the cogs spinning again.

It is important to state that knowing someone's SNPs does not tell you if a gene is switched "on" and expressing. Pairing the genetic report with functional lab testing and symptomatology can help determine if a SNP is expressing and, if so, to what degree.

APPENDIX 4B

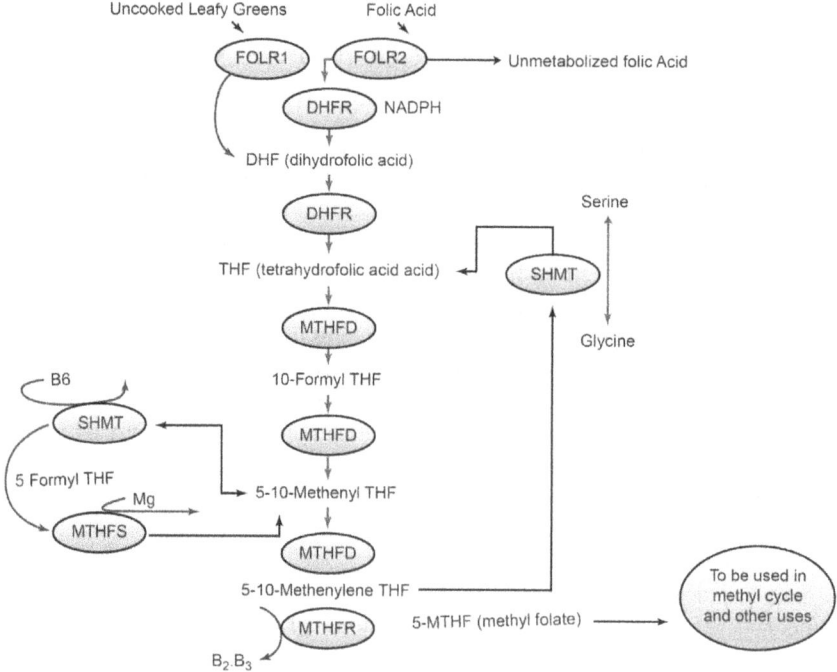

FIGURE 3 APPENDIX 4B   Genes involved in the methylation pathway.

Source: Image used with permission from NutriGenetic Research Institute

There are other genes in the methylation pathway that can be variated and, when combined with an MTHFR variant, can make the conversion efficiency of folic acid into methylfolate even worse (compounded even further by nutrient deficiencies). Some of these have been associated with neural tube defects (Parle-McDermott et al. 2006) and pregnancy loss (Figure 3 Appendix 4B).

These are:

- DHFR – produces a key enzyme in folate metabolism as it converts dihydrofolate into tetrahydrofolate, which are precursors to methylenetetrahydrofolate (MTHF). The DHFR enzyme also has another essential role in converting BH2 back into BH4, a vital cofactor involved in making nitric oxide (necessary for fertility), serotonin, and dopamine.
- FOLR – helps regulate folate transport into the cells
- MTHFD – catalyzes three reactions involving the interconversion of folate. May be related to endometriosis-associated infertility as well as susceptibility to miscarriage.
- SHMT – catalyzes tetrahydrofolate into 5,10-methylenetetrahydrofolate as well as the reversible conversion of serine into glycine. Glycine is one of the three amino acids that make up glutathione.

Genetic polymorphisms in any of these genes can alter outcomes, some of which can be problematic in more than just the methylation pathway.

APPENDIX 4C: WHY WE SHOULD NOT START SUPPLEMENTING WITH METHYLFOLATE WITHOUT MAKING SURE OTHER IMPORTANT FOUNDATIONS ARE IN PLACE

First, if your vitamin B12 levels are low and you start supplementing with high doses of methylfolate, something called "methyl trapping" can occur. Methyl trapping is problematic because methylfolate can't work without cobalamin (B12). The folate isn't properly utilized, and serum folate rises while intracellular (inside the cell) folate levels suffer. This is where only testing for serum folate and B12 levels can be misleading. Levels may look normal or even high, but this is because they are getting stuck in the blood and not getting into the cell to be used. If you want to check your methylation status, asking your practitioner or doctor to run a full panel, like a meth-ylation plasma profile (through Doctor's Data or Genova Laboratories) is the way to see much more of the pathway to know where wrenches might be.

Second, taking methylfolate while having low glutathione levels can make you more inflamed. Glutathione is considered the body's "master antioxidant" because

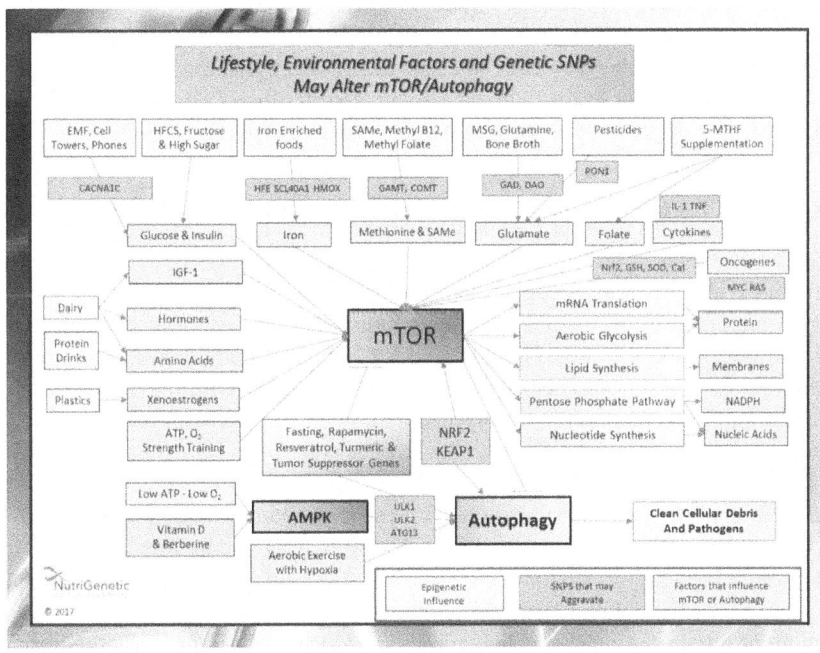

FIGURE 4 APPENDIX 4C   mTOR chart. Promoters and inhibitors of mTOR. Genetic SNPs and lifestyle and environmental factors that may affect the mTOR/autophagy balance.

Source: Reprinted with permission from NutriGenetic Research Institute

it can regenerate itself and other antioxidants. It's essential for detoxification and preventing oxidative stress. Stimulating methylation will spur detoxification, and if detox abilities or pathways are not up to snuff, this can cause problems if the body isn't able to adequately deal with the toxins that are stirred up. This is because if you are low in glutathione and start taking methylfolate, you stimulate phase 1 liver detox, and that creates toxins that have to be cleared by phase 2, which involves glutathione. If there isn't enough glutathione, things will get backed up and create inflammation.

Phase 1 detox is when the liver takes fat-soluble compounds (toxins) and transforms them into reactive intermediates with the help of the cytochrome P450 (CYP) enzymes made by an array of CYP genes. In phase 2, these intermediates are bound to substances like methyl groups (methylation), sulfur groups (sulfation/sulfonation), and acetyl groups (acetylation), which help them turn water soluble so they can be easily excreted in the feces (via bile) and urine. Phase 3 is the elimination of these toxins from the body. I discuss the three phases of detoxification in Chapter 12.

Third, methylfolate promotes something called mTOR, which stands for mammalian target of rapamycin. It's also known as mechanistic target of rapamycin, either of which sounds pretty badass, right? In short, mTOR plays an essential role in the regulation of normal cell growth, metabolism, and survival (Keppler-Noreuil et al. 2016). Disorders in mTOR are expansive, including autism, bipolar disorder, various cancers, and a range of growth abnormalities. This is obviously a necessary mechanism (especially during pregnancy), but when there are so many other factors that also promote cellular growth (see Figure 4 Appendix 4C), such as dairy (cow's milk is designed to grow a 1,200-pound cow), pesticides, iron-enriched foods, and sugar, the growth becomes aberrant and can cause things like cysts, tumors, endometriosis, stones, fibroids, etc. These absolutely mess with your fertility. Competent mTOR function is crucially important to your health and reproductive ability. So what can we do?

PROMOTION OF AUTOPHAGY TO KEEP MTOR IN CHECK

We need to balance cellular growth with autophagy, which is cellular cleanup. Autophagy literally translates to "self-eating." When the cell doesn't have any growth factors coming in, it starts to consume its less desirable damaged parts (cellular debris), improving efficiency, which helps the body detoxify, repair, and regenerate itself. This tampers down inflammation and optimizes the biological functioning of the body. This is why fasting can be so beneficial to the body. It is important to note that the body cannot be in a state of mTOR and autophagy at the same time.

mTOR dominance can be signified by the characteristics of aberrant growth but also by symptoms of weakened autophagy like age spots (a.k.a. liver spots) and poor detoxification. If someone with weakened autophagy/mTOR dominance starts supplementing with folate, this can further impede autophagy potential, creating more inflammation (and likely anxiety), which will scream for glutathione's help to put out the fire, leading us back to what I just mentioned about low glutathione levels.

ACTION STEPS

A few things you can do to support autophagy are:

- Ease into intermittent fasting. Start with a 12-hour window for fasting, then slowly increase that window of time.
- Moderate aerobic exercise (as opposed to strength training). Find the amount of exercise that doesn't leave you exhausted or irritable an hour or two later.
- Pulse the supplementation of resveratrol and/or berberine. I describe pulsing just ahead, but taking these two plant compounds can support autophagy. But we don't want to be in autophagy all the time. We still need cellular growth/mTOR, so pulsing these a few days per week may be ideal.

Note that a synergistic effect will take place if done in conjunction with one another.

To really maximize autophagy capabilities, I recommend pulsing supplements and foods that promote mTOR. For example, lots of people take L-glutamine and bone broth for gut healing, but as you can see in the chart, those substances promote mTOR. If, for example, you are fasting for a day but take L-glutamine or folate supplements that promote mTOR, you may be weakening your autophagy potential and negating the effects of fasting.

REFERENCES

Keppler-Noreuil, Kim M., Victoria E. R. Parker, Thomas N. Darling, and Julian A. Martinez-Agosto. 2016. "Somatic overgrowth disorders of the PI3K/AKT/mTOR pathway & therapeutic strategies." *American Journal of Medical Genetics Part C: Seminars in Medical Genetics* 172, no. 4, 402–421.

Klosin, Adam, Eduard Casas, Cristina Hidalgo-Carcedo, Tanya Vavouri, and Ben Lehner. 2017. "Transgenerational transmission of environmental information in C. elegans." *Science* 356, no. 6335, 320–323. https://science.sciencemag.org/content/356/6335/320.

Max-Planck-Gesellschaft. 2017. *Epigenetics between the generations: we inherit more than just genes.* www.sciencedaily.com/releases/2017/07/170717100548.htm.

Parle-McDermott, Anne, Peadar N. Kirke, James L. Mills, Anne M. Molloy, Christopher Cox, Valerie B. O'Leary, Faith Pangilinan, et al. 2006. "Confirmation of the R653Q polymorphism of the trifunctional C1-synthase enzyme as a maternal risk for neural tube defects in the Irish population." *European Journal of Human Genetics* 14, no. 6, 768–772.

Appendix 8

APPENDIX 8A: THE FENTON REACTION

The Fenton reaction occurs when hydrogen peroxide combines with free (unbound) iron and/or copper and creates hydroxyl radicals (a type of free radical). Hydrogen peroxide is a necessary substance produced by the body and beneficial only when not in excess. Hydroxyl radicals are very nasty free radicals that cause inflammation and damage cell structures, lipids, proteins, and DNA.

APPENDIX 8B: CERULOPLASMIN

Ceruloplasmin is the main copper-binding protein (Linder 2021) (metallothionein is the other) that helps get copper absorbed and delivered into the cells where it needs to be for the mitochondria to make ATP so iron can do its thing. If ceruloplasmin is low, free copper can rise, generating free radicals and damaging cells and tissues via oxidative stress from the Fenton reaction. This is how someone can be both copper deficient and copper toxic at the same time: the copper is getting stuck in the wrong places, creating inflammation, and is not getting to the right places. This will show up on testing as normal or even low copper in the serum, but high copper on a hair tissue mineral analysis (HTMA). Minerals and heavy metals get stored in tissue, but it would be a really invasive and painful test to gouge out some tissue for testing. Luckily, the hair is another place that minerals and toxins get stored, as hair is considered an excretory tissue. Although all methods have their pros and cons, HTMA can oftentimes be the preferred testing method for a few reasons:

1. As with iron, copper levels can look normal or even low in the blood, so this can be misleading if the copper is being sequestered in the tissues where it's accumulating and creating toxicity.
2. The body and blood are all about maintaining homeostasis. Blood is essentially just an oxygen and nutrient transporter into the tissues and CO_2 exporter out of the tissues. If the blood becomes deficient in calcium, for example, calcium will be pulled out of storage from the tissues and bones to be used, and so the blood levels may look normal while the body is essentially "robbing Peter to pay Paul" while the tissues and bones become depleted.
3. Blood levels can fluctuate daily, so if you were to test numerous days in a row, results could vary.

I recommend measuring blood markers (serum copper, ceruloplasmin, plasma zinc, serum iron, ferritin, and TIBC) along with an HTMA to get a more comprehensive look at what might be going on with iron and copper levels.

Beta carotene is considered vitamin A, but it is actually a precursor to vitamin A. It must be converted by the BCMO1 enzyme (made by the BCMO1 gene) into retinol for the body to be able to use it. Beta carotene is found in plants like leafy greens and orange vegetables while vitamin A is found in animal products like beef liver, eggs, and dairy products.

So what happens if you have variants in your BCMO1 gene? It's possible that your conversion rate is compromised. This is why everyone truly requires different amounts of each nutrient. You could be getting the same amount of beta carotene as your partner, but you could have an insufficient vitamin A level while theirs is optimal.

Ceruloplasmin is made in the liver at the command of the adrenals, so healthy adrenal functioning is a key component of optimal ceruloplasmin levels. Since the liver is essential to producing ceruloplasmin and processing excess and unbound copper, keeping it from being overwhelmed or sluggish is imperative.

APPENDIX 8C: THE HFE GENE

The HFE gene is often the only gene that is looked at when doctors are diagnosing hemochromatosis. While hemochromatosis is usually diagnosed by having homozygous variants on three HFE SNPs (rs1800562, rs1799945, and rs1800730) (Katsarou et al. 2019), heterozygous variants can still cause someone to absorb more than the body can effectively utilize.

Heterozygous HFE variants coupled with numerous other iron- and copper-related genes are why someone does not need to have a hemochromatosis diagnosis in order to have a problem with excess iron stores in the body.

THERE ARE OTHER GENES RELATING TO IRON DYSREGULATION BESIDES THE HFE GENE

First, there are the genes relating to copper. I already mentioned the BCMO1 gene, which is a cofactor in copper binding. There are numerous genes involved with copper binding and transport into and out of various cells, which I mention later. By the way, not all genetic tests include all the genes I mention in this book. You'll want to inquire about these before choosing a genetic test kit.

- SLC31A1 and SLC31A2 – Involved with copper transport. Variants here can lead to the potential for less-than-optimal copper transport and, therefore, diminished ceruloplasmin activity and iron utilization.
- ATOX (antioxidant protein 1) – Variants here can leave us more vulnerable to reactive oxygen species (ROS), resulting in a higher inflammatory burden. ATOX1 binds free metals like copper and prevents generation of ROS. It also delivers copper from cytosol to the ATPase transporters, ATP7A and ATP7B, both of which require ATOX1 to be functional. Without a functional ATOX1, we may have derangement and displacement of copper, which can result in low ceruloplasmin.
- ATP7A – Gets copper into the blood.

- ATP7B – Gets copper out of the liver.
- CP – This is the gene that provides instruction for making ceruloplasmin. Mutations in this gene cause aceruloplasminemia, which results in iron accumulation and tissue damage.

Outside the copper-related genes, there are a few genes that are involved with iron dysregulation besides the HFE gene.

- TMPRSS6 – associated with decreased serum ferritin and hemoglobin levels and iron deficiency anemia (Benyamin et al. 2009). This SNP has also been shown to modify the impact of HFE variants and may be protective against excess iron in individuals with HFE variants (Valenti et al. 2012). Variants in this gene may actually protect against hereditary hemochromatosis.
- SLC48A1 SNPs – These can result in poor gut absorption of iron, leading to anemia. Variants in SLC48A1 can offset HFE SNPS. Low hematocrit and low hemoglobin are often seen with SLC48A1 SNPs. Consider transdermal iron to bypass the gut and the need for iron infusions.
- The SLC40A1 gene contains instructions for making ferroportin. Ferroportin is the sole iron exporter in mammalian cells (Kasai et al. 2018) and plays a role in the metabolism of iron (Maio et al. 2021). Having variants in the SLC40A1 gene may cause some people to have trouble with iron getting stuck inside the cell, creating damage. With SLC40A1 variants, you are more likely to see low iron in blood work because iron may not be moving from the intestine into the blood. When this genetic variant occurs with one or more HFE variants, this can cause over-absorption of iron, and you can bet there's a good chance chronic inflammation will be present.
- The HMOX gene is a gene that makes the heme oxygenase enzyme that breaks down heme to make carbon monoxide and biliverdin. Biliverdin converts to bilirubin, which is an antioxidant that is especially helpful with lipid peroxidation. Variants in the HMOX gene will cause iron to oxidize via the Fenton reaction, creating inflammation. Sometimes with HMOX variants you'll see elevated hemoglobin because HMOX is not converting it. You may also see low biliverdin if HMOX is not converting heme.

APPENDIX 8D: IN ADDITION TO IMPROVING CERULOPLASMIN LEVELS TO IMPROVE THE UTILIZATION OF IRON, WE CAN ALSO REDUCE FENTON REACTION POTENTIAL BY REDUCING HYDROGEN PEROXIDE

Here are a few of the substances that research has shown to be effective in reducing hydrogen peroxide (H_2O_2) in the body:

- Catalase is an antioxidant enzyme produced by the body (the CAT gene) that helps turn hydrogen peroxide into water. Selenium is a cofactor for this reaction. Variants on your CAT gene or a deficiency in selenium from genetic predisposition, insufficient intake, or impaired absorption can be contributing factors for inflammation. Catalase is available in supplement form.

- Not necessarily an outright H_2O_2-lowering substance, but molecular hydrogen (H_2) in the form of hydrogen tablets or inhalation devices can help decrease hydroxyl radicals. Hydroxyl radicals are formed when hydrogen peroxide combines with free iron and/or copper in the Fenton reaction. Molecular hydrogen doesn't necessarily prevent the hydroxyl radicals from forming, but it can help neutralize them via electron donation, turning the hydroxyl radical ($\cdot$OH) into H2O once they have formed (Ohsawa et al. 2007).

REFERENCES

Benyamin, Beben, Manuel A. R. Ferreira, Gonneke Willemsen, Scott Gordon, Rita P. S. Middelberg, Brian P. McEvoy, Jouke-Jan Hottenga, et al. 2009. "Common variants in TMPRSS6 are associated with iron status and erythrocyte volume." *Nature Genetics* 41, no. 11, 1173–1175.

Kasai, Shuya, Junsei Mimura, Taku Ozaki, and Ken Itoh. 2018. "Emerging regulatory role of Nrf2 in iron, heme, and hemoglobin metabolism in physiology and disease." *Frontiers in Veterinary Science* 242.

Katsarou, Martha-Spyridoula, Maria Papasavva, Rozana Latsi, and Nikolaos Drakoulis. 2019. "Hemochromatosis: hereditary hemochromatosis and HFE gene." *Vitamins and Hormones* 110, 201–222.

Linder, Maria C. 2021. "Apoceruloplasmin: abundance, detection, formation, and metabolism." *Biomedicines* 9, no. 3, 233.

Maio, Nunziata, De-Liang Zhang, Manik C. Ghosh, Anshika Jain, Anna M. SantaMaria, and Tracey A. Rouault. 2021. "Mechanisms of cellular iron sensing, regulation of erythropoiesis and mitochondrial iron utilization." *In Seminars in Hematology* 58, no. 3, 161–174.

Ohsawa, Ikuroh, Masahiro Ishikawa, Kumiko Takahashi, Megumi Watanabe, Kiyomi Nishimaki, Kumi Yamagata, Ken-ichiro Katsura, Yasuo Katayama, Sadamitsu Asoh, and Shigeo Ohta. 2007. "Hydrogen acts as a therapeutic antioxidant by selectively reducing cytotoxic oxygen radicals." *Nature Medicine* 13, no. 6, 688–694.

Valenti, Luca, Anna Ludovica Fracanzani, Raffaela Rametta, Mirella Fraquelli, Giulia Soverini, Serena Pelusi, Paola Dongiovanni, Dario Conte, and Silvia Fargion. 2012. "Effect of the A736V TMPRSS6 polymorphism on the penetrance and clinical expression of hereditary hemochromatosis." *Journal of Hepatology* 57, no. 6, 1319–1325.

Appendix 9

APPENDIX 9A: DHEA

DHEA, a major precursor to steroid sex hormones, needs to be sulfated (have a sulfur group added to it). Almost all the DHEA circulating in the bloodstream is in the storage form of DHEA-S (DHEA Sulfate) and is the most abundant steroidal hormone in the body. The SULT2A1 gene controls DHEA sulfonation, turning DHEA into DHEA-S, and may have an influence on the body's ability to make this happen. There are other reasons DHEA may not be properly sulfated, including inflammation, sulfur- or oxalate-related SNPs, and just plain not getting enough in the diet.

Although excess levels of DHEA-S have been associated with polycystic ovary syndrome (PCOS), if DHEA is not properly sulfated, it leaves more DHEA to travel down the path towards androgen production, causing hair loss, facial hair, acne, and everyone's favorite, easy irritation. If this is the case, we can do some Band-Aid approaches to help lessen the androgen symptoms, like nettles, reishi mushroom, and EGCG (green tea is a rich source), but we still want to get to the cause of the problem.

Side note on PCOS: In animal and human studies, it has been shown that androgens appear to have a boosting effect on urinary stone formation. Hyperandrogenism, the main feature of PCOS, may trigger the urinary stone formation (Kaygusuz et al. 2013).

Aromatase is an enzyme that converts testosterone into estrogen, and excess inflammation upregulates aromatase. Oxalates cause inflammation that upregulates aromatase, elevating estrogen and leading to estrogen-dominant issues like fibroids and endometriosis. To add insult to injury, oxalates will also rob the body of the sulfur molecule that is needed for hormonal balance, and when we don't have enough sulfur, our hormones will swing wildly.

Oxalates cause inflammation and oxidative stress. They also make it harder for the body to combat that oxidative stress because when they dominate, the sulfate needed to make superstar-antioxidant glutathione is depleted, which causes more oxidative stress and poor detoxification of hormones and xenoestrogens. Yet another vicious cycle . . .

APPENDIX 9B: OXALATE-RELATED GENES (NOT INCLUDING SULFATION GENES) AND SECONDARY HYPEROXALURIA

- The GRHPR gene provides instructions for making an enzyme that makes glyoxylate and hydroxypyruvate reductase (Medicine n.d.). This enzyme plays a role in preventing the buildup of glyoxylate by converting it into glycolate. Glycolate can be easily eliminated from the body. Although variants here can decrease the conversion rate and cause a buildup of glyoxylate, it may only be an issue with homozygous variants, as having heterozygous variants will likely not cause noteworthy issues with oxalates.

- The HOGA1 gene codes for making the 4-hydroxy-2-oxoglutarate aldolase (HOGA) enzyme. This enzyme is found in liver and kidney cells, specifically in the mitochondria, the energy-producing centers in cells (National Library of Medicine, n.d.-c). Variations in the gene may lead to hyperoxaluria type 3. Typically, in my experience (and that of my colleagues and the current 50,000 people in the Functional Genomic Analysis software), for it to be much of an issue, variants in the HOGA1 gene generally need to be homozygous. Keep in mind that having several heterozygous variants, coupled with variants in the other oxalate genes, can compound the predisposition.
- The AGXT gene appears to be the most significantly related to oxalate issues (Xu et al. 2021) (Mandrile et al. 2014), especially if there are homozygous variants, as these people have an increased likelihood of having issues with kidney stones. With the other oxalate-related genes, oxalates can aggregate in any tissue, and people with these variants are rarely kidney stone formers. But AGXT can increase the likelihood of kidney stone formation, although less than 1% of oxalate issues present with kidney stones. Most presentations are in the form of pain, when oxalates are trapped in the body and can create some serious health conditions. And unfortunately, only a heterozygous variant can be enough to cause oxalate issues. This gene is the most researched oxalate-related gene in the medical community and primary type 1 hyperoxaluria.
- The SPP1 gene is involved in the attachment of osteoclasts (cells that break down bone and are responsible for bone resorption) to the mineralized bone matrix (National Library of Medicine, n.d.-a). What that means in terms of oxalates is when you have SPP1 variants, it's harder for calcium to attach to the bone matrix and easier for the oxalate to grab on to it and form oxalate crystals.

Secondary hyperoxaluria is the effect of various influences that cause oxalates to be more elevated than the body can effectively clear. Having variants in the HOGA1, AGXT, and GRHPR genes definitely contribute to fueling this fire. Issues with oxalates are, in part, due to microbiome imbalance and a lack of the bacteria that breaks it down. The Great Plains Laboratory website states

> Candida and Aspergillus species can produce oxalates. These species have certain enzymes that allow them to use glyoxylate as a means of making energy (it is an intermediate in their Tricarboxylic Acid (TCA) or Krebs cycle). Individuals with elevations in Candida or Aspergillus frequently have a subsequent elevation in oxalate metabolites. The degree of elevation may or may not be proportional to the yeast/mold overgrowth.
>
> (Bonovich 2016)

APPENDIX 9C: A QUICK NOTE ON MAST
CELL ACTIVATION AND OXALATES

This connection is a two-way street, since oxalates can trigger mast cell activation (O'Hara n.d.). Mast cells can create intestinal permeability, allowing us to over-absorb oxalates and other substances (e.g., undigested proteins) that shouldn't be absorbed.

When oxalates signal the mast cells to activate, the downstream potential consequences are numerous, including histamine release (which triggers mast cell activation, and around the cycle goes), leading to histamine intolerance, which has been tied to mast cell activation syndrome and Ehlers-Danlos syndrome. (This is huge; so many people suffer from MCAS and EDS, many without even being aware of it!)

WHAT A URINE ORGANIC ACID TEST
CAN TELL US ABOUT OXALATES

My most recommended test by far is the urine organic acid test (OAT) by Great Plains Laboratory. This test has three direct markers for oxalates as well as a few other markers that can indicate (or commonly occur with) excess oxalates in the body. The first two, glyceric and glycolic, are typically related to genetic predisposition and will likely need long-term support if elevated. Additionally, glyceric elevations can indicate that GRHPR variants may be expressing, and glycolic acid will get higher and worsen as B6 levels go lower.

The third marker is oxalic acid, and that typically reflects secondary or consequential reasons for oxalate issues, like excess consumption of oxalates (green smoothies every day or eating more almond flour products because of a gluten-free diet), fat malabsorption, low vitamin B6 levels, or yeast and/or fungal overgrowth. Elevated oxalic acid may be associated with dysbiosis from *Aspergillus*, *Penicillium*, and possibly candida or from high doses of vitamin C.

Yeast and fungal markers on the first page can be an indicator that oxalates may be a problem since certain yeast and fungi can produce oxalates. However, low or normal levels of yeast and fungal markers do not signify that oxalates are not a problem and could be related to other factors. If yeast or fungal markers are elevated, antifungal therapy may reduce oxalates. These markers are more likely to be elevated if someone has a history of mold exposure. (Read Chapter 7.)

Citrate levels that trend on the lower side can point to oxalate issues. I mentioned the citrate form of minerals in the recommendation list earlier since citrate helps lower oxalates. Oxalates can be made endogenously in the citric acid cycle. Low citrate has been associated with spontaneous kidney stone formation (Zuckerman and Assimos 2009).

Pyridoxic acid is a major metabolite of vitamin B6. As stated earlier, B6 is an integral factor in oxalate metabolism, and when it is low, there can be oxalate issues.

If oxalate levels are low or normal on an OAT, it does not necessarily mean that oxalates are not an issue. As with heavy metal testing, some peoples' bodies are very good at sequestering substances or "sweeping them under the rug." The test only reflects what is being eliminated from the body, so if markers look normal, act based on symptoms or other indicative markers. It is a good idea to retest after a lower-oxalate diet and other oxalate support have been implemented.

As I stated in Chapter 2, I am extremely well versed in the interpretation of the urine organic acids test, far beyond what is stated in the interpretation that comes with test results. I have researched and studied each marker, and this test has been a common topic of discussion in the functional medicine mastermind group of practitioners that I have been a member of. I am available for one-to-one consultations to interpret your or your patients' organic acid test results, in addition to consults for genomic interpretations. Please contact me to learn more: info@JaclynDowns.com.

REFERENCES

Bonovich, Jessica, RN. 2016. *Oxalates*, August 8. www.greatplainslaboratory.com/gpl-blog-source/tag/Jessica+Bonovich+RN+BSN.

Kaygusuz, Ikbal, Omer Faruk Karatas, Hasan Kafali, Ersin Cimentepe, and Dogan Unal. 2013. "Is polycystic ovarian syndrome a risk factor for urolithiasis?" *Urolithiasis* 41, no. 4, 361–362.

Mandrile, Giorgia, Christiaan S. Van Woerden, Paola Berchialla, Bodo B. Beck, Cécile Acquaviva Bourdain, Sally-Anne Hulton, Gill Rumsby, and OxalEurope Consortium. 2014. "Data from a large European study indicate that the outcome of primary hyperoxaluria type 1 correlates with the AGXT mutation type." *Kidney International* 86, no. 6, 1197–1204.

National Library of Medicine. n.d.-a. *Genetic Testing Registry SPP1 secreted phosphoprotein 1*. www.ncbi.nlm.nih.gov/gtr/genes/6696/.

National Library of Medicine. n.d.-b. *GRHPR gene*. https://medlineplus.gov/genetics/gene/grhpr/.

National Library of Medicine. n.d.-c. *HOGA1 gene*. https://medlineplus.gov/genetics/gene/hoga1/.

O'Hara, Beth. n.d. *Oxalates and the mast cell activation syndrome | histamine intolerance connection.* https://mastcell360.com/oxalates-and-the-mast-cell-activation-syndrome-istamine-ntolerance-connection/.

Xu, Chang Bao, Xu Dong Zhou, Hong En Xu, Yong Li Zhao, Xing Hua Zhao, Dan Hua Liu, Yong An Tian, et al. 2021. "A novel nonsense variant of the AGXT identified in a Chinese family: special variant research in the Chinese reference genome." *BMC Nephrology* 22, no. 1, 1–8.

Zuckerman, Jack M., and Dean G. Assimos. 2009. "Hypocitraturia: pathophysiology and medical management." *Reviews in Urology* 11, no. 3, 134.

Appendix 10

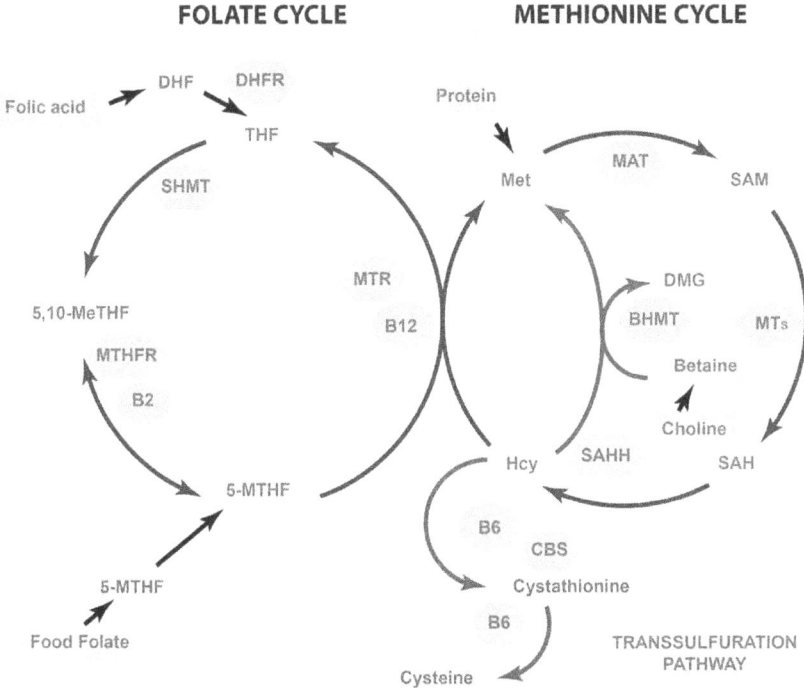

FIGURE 1 APPENDIX 10 Choline is a main player in the methylation pathway, and its levels are dependent on PEMT and BHMT activity. More specifically, choline is the precursor of betaine, which provides a methyl group needed to convert homocysteine to methionine via the enzyme betaine-homocysteine methyltransferase, made by the BHMT gene. Methionine makes SAMe, the universal methyl donor needed for methylation.

Appendix 11

Over the past few years, the research team at the NutriGenetic Research Institute has come across many topics that we were/are convinced are root causes of many, if not most, illnesses, of which insufficient antioxidant activity and iron dysregulation are two. While they certainly play huge roles in metabolic balance (or lack thereof), it wasn't until we came across the NOX enzyme that we perfectly tied all those previous topics together.

Before I go into what NOX (NADPH oxidase) is and does, it is important to discuss what NADPH is first.

We are (w)holistic beings. Our current medical system compartmentalizes different systems in the body, with each doctor having their own specialty, which is one reason why root causes are rarely addressed. Everything is connected in the body. One of the things my dad taught me early on, using a musical metaphor, is that "the entire orchestra of nutrition is required to play the symphony of biology." I often tell my clients that magnesium, histamine, and/or blood sugar regulation ability have their fingers in many pots in the body because they are used in so many reactions and because there are a plethora of downstream effects if they are imbalanced. There are many other nutrients and substances that have pervasive downstream effects as well, especially NADPH.

NADPH stands for nicotinamide adenine dinucleotide phosphate. It is an essential electron donor in all organisms. This can get really complex, really quickly. There are so many things I could write relating to NADPH, but I'll stick with relevance to fertility and promise not to get too complex and dry.

NADPH is most definitely a super-ubiquitous (supiquitous!) molecule that is used for extremely critical functions in the body. These include:

- Antioxidant production
- Reducing agent that donates electrons – What this means is that it recycles/ recharges antioxidants back into usable forms once they've neutralized a substance.
- DNA synthesis and repair
- Chromosomal integrity
- Epigenetic modifications
- Energy production
- Balance of mTOR and autophagy
- Supporting sirtuins (the longevity genes)
- Detoxification (including hormone-disrupting xenobiotics)
- Making steroid hormones (including cortisol and reproductive hormones)
- Lipid synthesis (needed for sex and stress hormone balance)
- Mitochondrial functioning
- Protecting the immune system
- Protecting red blood cells
- Cellular balance and regrowth

- Folate utilization
- Gene expression
- Aging/anti-aging

And finally, NADPH is essential for nitric oxide (NO) production. Nitric oxide was the topic of the 1998 Nobel Prize winner, and it has been dubbed "Molecule of the Year" because it is such a ubiquitous and vital substance. Many studies have declared that nitric oxide is crucial for fertility, as it promotes healthy cervical mucus, egg health (American Chemical Society 2005), and implantation (Mörlin et al. 2005).

Nerd note: For those of you who are about to get all excited about boosting your nitric oxide: A cautionary note about supplementing with L-arginine to boost nitric oxide.

The amino acid L-arginine is most known for its role in converting to nitric oxide. Many people buy this inexpensive supplement specifically for this purpose, but there are a few important points to consider beforehand.

Anyone with any type of herpes viral load, even when dormant, may have issues from arginine, as arginine agitates the herpes virus by exacerbating/increasing its virulent replication (Becker et al. 1967).

Also, a really cool substance called BH4 (the scientific abbreviation for tetrahydrobiopterin) is needed in good amounts to combine with arginine to form nitric oxide. If you don't have enough BH4 because of genetic variants related to its production or recycling (which include DHFR, QDPR, and GCH1 genes) or if it is being used up by other processes that it is required for (like neurotransmitter production and keeping ammonia levels in check), then arginine won't get turned into nitric oxide. Instead, something called NOS uncoupling can occur and create a boatload of oxidative stress and inflammation.

If you do want to boost your nitric oxide, Zach Bush has some videos on a quick and easy exercise routine (four minutes, y'all!) that boosts your NO levels, called the Nitric Oxide Dump.

As you can see in the bullet points, if any of these factors are compromised, the downstream effects can be numerous and very detrimental.

NADPH IS REQUIRED FOR GLUTATHIONE RECYCLING

NADPH converts oxidized glutathione back into reduced glutathione (the master antioxidant) with the help of riboflavin (vitamin B2). In some instances, supplementing with glutathione causes people to feel very ill or inflamed after a dosage. It is usually chalked up to a Herxheimer (detox) reaction, but this may not be the case. It may be that NADPH levels are low, and the glutathione isn't able to get recycled (glutathione recycling is also governed by the GSR gene), staying stuck in its oxidized form, creating inflammation, and hindering detoxification. If this is the case, supplementing with it only pours gasoline on the fire. While glutathione is an extremely important and beneficial antioxidant, there are times and situations where it is not always ideal, or at least, not yet.

NOW, ON TO NOX

NADPH also has another important job: signaling reactive oxygen species (ROS), a type of free radical. NADPH fuels an enzyme called NADPH oxidase (NOX). As far as current research shows, NOX's only job is to create free radicals to make enough inflammation to kill off pathogens. Inflammation is not always a bad thing; it is only bad when it is excessive and/or chronic.

Mice that had been bred to have the NOX gene knocked out (removed) quickly died because their immune systems couldn't fight off pathogens. So, while we need NADPH to fuel NOX, it needs to be in just the right amount so it doesn't create too much inflammation (which has been referred to as the "Goldilocks zone") (Alleman et al. 2014).

When the NOX enzyme is overstimulated by epigenetic factors, this leads to the "NADPH steal," a term my colleague, Bob Miller, coined. This means that instead of NADPH contributing to all the wonderful things that it is needed for, it is shuttled towards the NOX enzyme to "put out fires."

Studies have found that NOX overactivity and, therefore, the free radicals it generates play a significant role in a wide range of chronic health conditions, including fertility issues. Several articles have detailed NOX's relationship with endometriosis, hormone synthesis, fertilization, sperm health and male infertility, and outcomes of IVF (Nassif et al. 2016; Krzastek et al. 2020).

One review article states that endometriosis induces decreased quantities of oocytes and embryos, decreased embryo quality, and decreased implantation and pregnancy rates in patients with endometriosis (Máté et al. 2018). It then goes on to discuss evidence that the reactive oxygen species (ROS) generated in endometriosis patients damages intracellular structures and genomic material, which adversely impacts the structural integrity and viability of oocytes, sperm, and embryos.

NOX MUST BE KEPT UNDER CONTROL

So, what stimulates NOX? Unfortunately, many things in our modern world fuel the NOX enzyme, which depletes NADPH's ability to fuel all the beneficial functions. Oxalates are one of those things (detailed in Chapter 9). Another is excessive iron, either caused by genetic predisposition (discussed in Chapter 8) or excessive intake of iron-fortified food and supplements. In Figure 1 Appendix 11A, the boxes with arrows pointing towards NOX are the things that promote NOX activity.

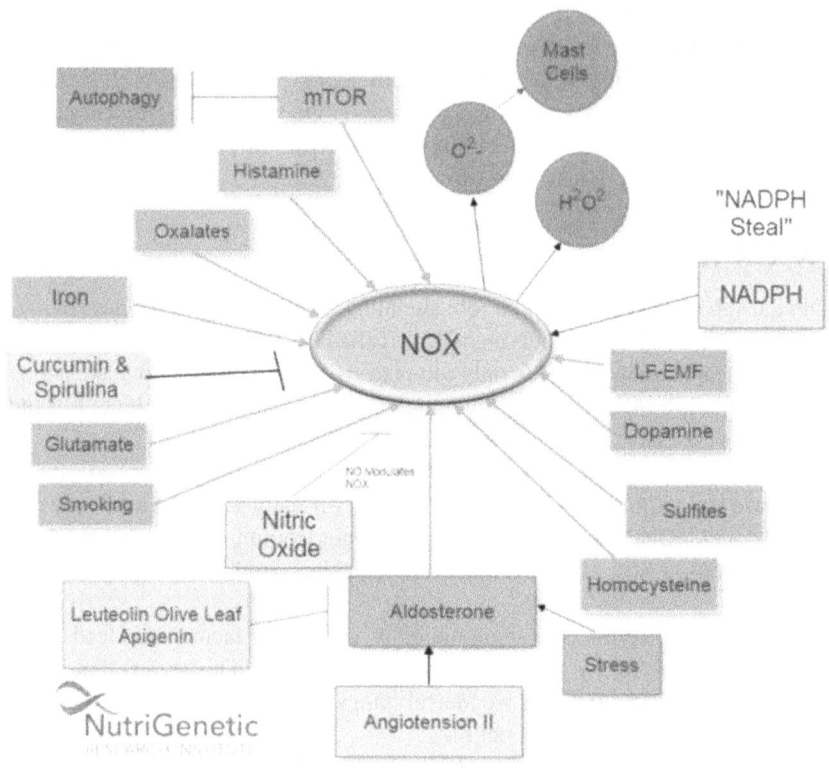

FIGURE 1 APPENDIX 11A   Factors known to promote or inhibit NOX activity.

Source: Used with permission from NutriGenetic Research Institute

Excessive NOX activation has the potential to lead to increased inflammation and, therefore, a decreased ability to metabolize environmental toxins. With higher NOX activity, there is less NADPH to fight free radicals, increasing the potential for them to oxidize and damage cell membranes, DNA, and other proteins. We must calm the things that stimulate the NOX enzyme (rectangles in Figure 1 Appendix 11A) so that our NADPH is not used up fueling NOX activity.

MTOR STIMULATES NOX

There is accumulating evidence that mTOR (discussed in Chapter 4) plays a significant role in the regulation of NOX. Thus, excessive stimulation of the mTOR pathway may also contribute to NOX stimulation and, subsequently, the production of free radicals (Eid et al. 2013). Refer back to the mTOR chart in Chapter 4 to see the things that stimulate mTOR.

HOMOCYSTEINE STIMULATES NOX

The NOX enzyme is also stimulated by elevated homocysteine. Elevated homo-cysteine levels have been associated with cardiovascular complications, miscar-riages, preeclampsia, birth defects, and neurodegenerative diseases (Pizzorno 2014).

However, homocysteine is not a bad guy. It can be considered a storage molecule for sulfur and is an important factor in the methylation and transsulfuration pathways, all of which I discussed previously. Homocysteine has a Goldilocks zone as well.

ADDITIONAL NERD NOTES ON HOMOCYSTEINE

Homocysteine is needed to make glutathione (GSH). Problems with recycling homocysteine back into methionine (the precursor to the universal methyl donor SAMe) can occur because of deficiencies in vitamins B6 or B12, folate, zinc, and/or choline and also because of SNPs in the MTR, MTRR, MTHFR, BHMT, and/or PEMT genes (Figure 2 Appendix 11A).

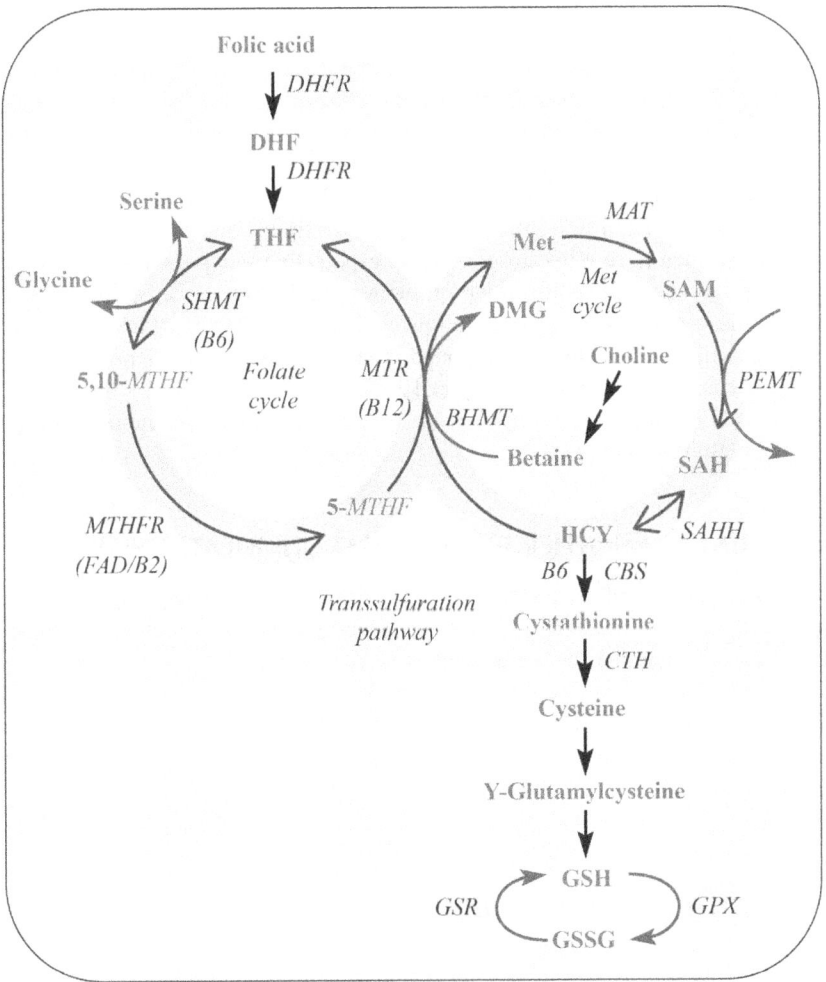

FIGURE 2 APPENDIX 11A Homocysteine (HCY) sits at the intersection of the methionine cycle and the transsulfuration pathway. The transsulfuration pathway's ultimate job is to turn homocysteine into glutathione. The methionine cycle's primary job is to make sure homocysteine is recycled back up into SAMe, which drives methylation.

- MTHFR – Converts folic acid into methylfolate.
- MTRR – Transfers the methyl group from methylfolate and attaches it to cobalamin (vitamin B12) to turn it into methylcobalamin. Because it puts a methyl group on B12, SNPs here may affect B12 levels.
- MTR – Uses methylfolate and methylcobalamin (vitamin B12) to convert homocysteine to methionine. Variants in this gene have been associated with an increased risk of birth defects that occur during the development of the brain and spinal cord (neural tube defects). Some studies have suggested that the variant also increases the risk of having a child with Down syndrome, but other studies found no increased risk (National Library Medicine n.d.).
- PEMT – Encodes an enzyme that converts phosphatidylethanolamine to phosphatidylcholine. It is the only producer of phosphatidylcholine in the body. People with PEMT variants, which are quite common, have increased need for choline, which must be acquired through external sources, either with choline or phosphatidylcholine supplementation or via sunflower lecithin. PEMT plays a big part in another pathway, or "backup route," for the body to ensure homocysteine gets recycled back into methionine.
  - On a related note, the PEMT gene is stimulated by estrogen. When women have low estrogen levels, especially menopausal women, they may develop gallbladder problems, intolerance to fats, SIBO, and issues losing weight due to low choline levels. Having PEMT variants will very well likely compound issues with phosphatidylcholine. I discussed this further in Chapter 10.
- BHMT – Supports homocysteine to methionine conversion. Supported with trimethylglycine.

HISTAMINE IS ANOTHER FACTOR THAT STIMULATES NOX

When histamine stimulates NOX, NOX then stimulates mast cells (immune cells that coordinate how the immune and nervous systems respond to various substances), which trigger histamine release as well as more inflammatory proteins, becoming a vicious cycle. The kicker here is that histamine and estrogen feed each other. This can be very bad news and lead to estrogen dominance and all the unpleasant things that come along with it. To learn more about histamine intolerance and clearance, refer to Chapter 16.

THE DUTCH TEST INCLUDES A MARKER
FOR OXIDATIVE STRESS

There is one test that actually measures the levels of your three estrogens (estrone, estradiol, and estriol) and shows how they are metabolizing. This is the DUTCH test, and it is the gold standard for hormone testing in functional medicine and functional nutrition. In addition to seeing how your estrogens are being metabolized, you can use it to see how they are being methylated. It also measures progesterone and testosterone metabolism, as well as cortisol production and utilization. It is one of the few tests that I am aware of that measures 8-OHDG, a direct measure of oxidative stress. It even measures a small number of organic acids. I have no affiliation with this test or laboratory; I just think it is such a great test for seeing a snapshot of what is currently happening with the hormones in your body.

Circling back around, if we don't clear histamine, we make NOX, which stimulates mast cells to create inflammation. The inflammation will cause glutathione to respond and work overtime to squelch the inflammation, depleting glutathione and hindering its ability to be recycled since the NADPH needed to recycle it is getting used to fuel NOX because it's trying to clear histamine instead of recycling antioxidants. This increases oxidative stress and compromises detoxification pathways. What a nasty cycle. Elevated histamine can cause much more trouble than itchy eyes.

GLUTAMATE STIMULATES NOX

Excess or improperly used glutamate stimulates NOX activity (Guemez-Gamboa et al. 2011), as well as anxiety and fatigue. However, there are numerous other ways that excess glutamate can create inflammation and vice versa.

Glutamate is an excitatory neurotransmitter that causes our brains to function quickly, which is great for cognitive functioning. Glutamate gets converted to the calming neurotransmitter gamma-aminobutyric acid (commonly called GABA), eliciting calmness, like the way you feel after a yoga class (because yoga promotes GABA). The glutamate-to-GABA conversion takes place via the GAD enzyme (made by the GAD gene) and must be strictly moderated for optimal function of the central nervous system. Inflammation hinders the glutamate-to-GABA conversion (so do lead, mercury, and aluminum), as does an insufficiency in vitamin B6, as B6 is a necessary cofactor for this conversion.

When inflammation, GAD variants, heavy metal toxicity, and/or B6 deficiency hinders this conversion, glutamate levels may rise, combined with an insufficient amount of GABA, which can trigger anxiety and/or easy agitation because the neurons are overstimulated by the excess glutamate.

Clinical pearl: ATP is required for glutamate-to-GABA conversion. Mitochondrial dysfunction causes ATP production to decrease, which affects the glutamate-to-GABA conversion. This excess glutamate can cause an inflammatory cascade and suppress the immune system.

NATURAL PROGESTERONE PROMOTES GABA AND SUPPRESSES GLUTAMATE

Excess glutamate is also the result of low progesterone levels, as progesterone enhances the GABA system, thereby protecting against excess glutamate. When progesterone is low, we may tend to be more anxious or easily irritated. Vitamin B6 is required for glutamate-to-GABA conversion and is also a precursor to progesterone. If you have good B6 levels that encourage healthy progesterone levels, then your chance of feeling pretty chill increases, which increases the likelihood for your body to be "pro-gestation."

CAVEAT FOR GABA SUPPLEMENTATION

I don't often recommend that my clients supplement with GABA unless their glutamate is low along with it, because it could actually make them more anxious and inflamed. Taking GABA can spare your glutamate to GABA conversion since your brain will see that there is now enough GABA and will slow conversion causing glutamate to be elevated. I tell my clients that I would rather their bodies make it than take it (supplement with it). Even excess GABA can directly suppress dopamine, the happiness, motivation, concentration, cravings control, and anti-stress neurotransmitter. Excess GABA has even been associated with suicidal ideation (Blum et al. 2012).

Glutamate is also converted to other metabolites, like glutamine, one of the precursors for glutathione production. Glutamate and glutamine actually interconvert ("bi-directional" metabolism). The GLUL gene makes the blueprint for glutamate to convert to glutamine. Variants here can hinder this conversion, causing anxiety or easy agitation due to elevated glutamate, as well as preventing downstream anti-inflammatory glutathione from being synthesized.

Glutamate is also needed for energy production. The glutamate dehydrogenase enzyme, made by the GLUD gene, supports the glutamate-to-alpha-ketoglutarate conversion that creates energy via the Krebs cycle, so if you have variants in GLUD, glutamate may not efficiently turn into cellular energy, which the body needs to be able to grow a baby. The glutamate that is not converted can get backed up, causing you to feel wired, tired, and anxious.

Circling back around to my statement that glutamate stimulates NOX; this is part of a nasty cycle because NOX creates inflammation, which uses precious glutathione in an attempt to put out the inflammatory fire. This inflammation hinders glutamate-to-GABA conversion, and around we go with elevated glutamate, anxiousness, and inflammation. Here's the crappy bonus: Glutamate stimulates mTOR as well, which I discussed in Chapter 4.

ACTION STEPS

Things that I personally use for healthy glutamate levels:

- Cannabinoids (CBD) help modulate glutamate and dopamine receptor sites, which is what makes them great for anxiety and insomnia. CBD also may activate GABA receptors, producing anxiolytic effects. CBD also helps with autonomic nervous system balance ("fight or flight" versus "rest, digest, repair, reproduce").

- Magnesium is critical for the proper physiological function of the gluta-mate receptor known as NMDAR. NMDA receptors are activated when glutamate binds to them. Research suggests magnesium has the ability to act as an antagonist and block NMDA receptors while it also functions as a GABA agonist. My favorite form to take orally is magnesium threonate and transdermally, Epsom salts.
- Honokiol acts to squelch glutamate by helping convert glutamate to GABA. During research in mice, honokiol exposure has also been correlated with increased GAD activity; similarly, during an in vitro mouse study, honokiol was shown to inhibit repetitive neural firing by blocking glutamate and the NMDA receptor (Woodbury et al. 2013).
- Pyridoxal-5-Phosphate (P5P), the active form of vitamin B6, enhances GAD activity because it is a cofactor for the GAD enzyme, which is respon-sible for the conversion of glutamate to GABA.
- Phosphatidylserine may regulate glutamate receptor activity and help calm down brain chatter.

Just a heads-up: NOX upregulation can also affect your offspring for years to come. Increased ROS production from the NOX2 enzyme is a possible molecular mecha-nism responsible for developmental origins of cardiovascular disease in the offspring of diabetic mothers (Zhang et al. 2018).

TAMP DOWN NOX ACTIVITY TO SPARE NADPH

As the aforementioned environmental factors stimulate NOX, NOX uses NADPH to try to put out inflammation. By tamping down the things that stimulate NOX, our bodies won't have to use so much NADPH to put out fires, leaving more available to recycle antioxidants. I feel that this is a key factor in optimizing fertility. If the body is preoccupied with trying to squelch inflammation, it is going to know that now is not a safe time to procreate.

NAD+ AND NADPH: NOT TO BE CONFUSED, BUT DEFINITELY RELATED

In doing research on NADPH, you'll absolutely learn about NAD (and its forms NAD+ and NADH). These are very popular topics in functional medicine cir-cles right now. NAD and NADPH can interconvert in the body as needed. The basic difference between the two is that NADPH possesses a phosphate, and its function lies more with cellular antioxidants and producing reactive oxygen species (via NOX), whereas NAD+ mediates energy production (ATP) and is imperative for healthy mitochondrial functioning. If we don't have NAD, we don't have healthy mitochondria. We need functioning mitochondria for healthy reproduction.

One study showed that reproductive aging in female mammals is an irreversible process associated with declining oocyte quality, which is the rate-limiting factor for fertility (Bertoldo et al. 2020). This study demonstrated that loss of oocyte quality with age accompanies declining levels of NAD+, and treatment with the NAD+ metabolic precursor nicotinamide mononucleotide (NMN) rejuvenates oocyte quality in aged animals, restoring fertility. The added bonus that was noted in this study is that NMN restores not only egg quality but also embryo development and functional fertility. This is huge!

This study also states that, in addition to NAD+, declining NADPH is associated with oocyte dysfunction during reproductive aging.

WHAT ARE NADH AND NAD+?

NADH stands for nicotinamide adenine dinucleotide. It is the reduced form of NAD+, a coenzyme found in all living cells. It is synthesized in the body from vitamin B3 (niacin or nicotinamide). NADH plays a key role in the production of energy through ATP generation.

NADH is generated from NAD+ in the citric acid cycle (a.k.a. the Krebs cycle or tricarboxylic acid cycle) that makes ATP. NAD is important for so many functions. It is critical to healthy aging and longevity, particularly for stimulating sirtuins (made by SIRT genes, known as our "longevity genes"), the DNA damage repair enzymes, and telomere maintenance (the 'tail' of our chromosomes). High NAD+ is necessary for healthy metabolism, mitochondria, and cell survival. Food intake, exercise, and even time of day affect NAD levels and activity. Low NAD+ can contribute to fatigue and several diseases. NAD+ levels decline with age, potentially altering metabolism and increasing susceptibility to disease.

One study even referred to NAD+ as an "Achilles heel" whose decline results in many age-associated pathologies (Imai and Guarente 2014). This study stated that NAD+ levels decline with aging and cause defects in the nucleus and mitochondria of cells. By now, Dear Reader, you know that optimal cellular functioning is needed for fertility, so you can grasp the importance of NAD+ for anyone trying to conceive and sustain a pregnancy.

ACTION STEPS FOR SUPPORTING NAD+ AND NADPH LEVELS

There are quite a few genes in the NAD+/NADH and NADP+/NADPH pathways. This is more complex than I want to write about in this book, but there are genetic reports and qualified practitioners (like myself – feel free to book a consult to help you interpret your genetics or those of your patients/clients) who can assist you with navigating the nuances of particular pathways. There are, however, some substances that can help support the pathways overall or that can be beneficial for certain steps along the pathways.

- B vitamins, especially vitamin B2, in the form of riboflavin-5-phosphate. NADPH, in concert with riboflavin, helps convert oxidized glutathione into its usable reduced form. I do not recommend taking isolated B vitamin supplements unless you are already taking a bioavailable B complex (forms that do not need to convert to a usable form and that are ready for the body to use). Taking a single B vitamin can affect levels of the other B vitamins, throwing them out of range. Your B vitamins should be taken with food or in a supplement made with a food matrix.

- Nicotinamide riboside (NR) and nicotinamide mononucleotide (NMN) are derivatives of niacin. Niacin is also known as vitamin B3 and comes in the form of nicotinic acid and/or nicotinamide/niacinamide. These are all precursors and intermediates to synthesize NAD and NADPH. All tissues in the body convert absorbed niacin into its primarily active form, NAD. Super ubiquitous (supiquitous!), more than 400 enzymatic reactions require NAD (National Institutes of Health n.d.). Many people don't like niacin supplements because of flushing, and most people flush long before they can get NAD+ levels up anyway. Large doses of no-flush niacin suppress sirtuin activity, so the preferred way is through nicotinamide riboside (NR) or nicotinamide mononucleotide (NMN), which support sirtuins and raise NAD+ and NADPH levels.
- Some plant compounds that have studies indicating potential inhibition of NOX activity are curcumin, luteolin, apigenin, olive leaf, and spirulina (Liwa et al. 2017).
- Molecular hydrogen (H_2) inhibits the NOX enzyme, stabilizes mast cells, and spares NAD and NADPH. As of now, I am aware of only one contraindication with hydrogen tablet supplementation, and that is with methane-driven SIBO. Archaea organisms feed on hydrogen, so when there is an overabundance of archaea, there will be a quick onset of symptoms from oral administration of hydrogen. Gas, bloating, brain fog, and fatigue can ensue; however, they are less likely with hydrogen inhalation devices.
- Supplementation aside, there are dietary and lifestyle things that can preserve or boost NADPH levels. Keeping healthy blood glucose levels and avoiding fructose are among them. Excess glucose is converted to fructose, which, in order to metabolize, will then require a molecule of NADPH to turn to a molecule of NADH, taking away from its antioxidant capabilities (Fessel and Oldham 2018). So, keeping your glucose at healthy levels (an ideal fasting glucose level is 85) and avoiding fructose are part of the equation.
- Other ways to raise your levels without supplementation are getting serious about your sleep and sleep hygiene, some forms of fasting, and moving your body in a loving way (walking, dance, HIIT, whatever you enjoy that makes you feel good and energized).

LET'S GO UPSTREAM OF NADPH

A note on a very important, very common genetic variant (1 in 16 people have it), glucose-6-phosphate dehydrogenase (G6PD): The G6PD gene codes for the glucose-6-phosphate dehydrogenase enzyme. It is the most common genetic abnormality, affecting an estimated 400 million people worldwide, according to the World Health Organization.

G6PD supplies the energy needed to produce NADPH. Red blood cells are the only type of cells that completely depend upon this pathway. The G6PD enzyme converts NADP+ into NADPH, so with G6PD deficiency, there is not enough NADPH. This makes red blood cells more susceptible to reactive oxygen species, which may cause anemia, spontaneous abortions, and problems with fetuses (Peters and Van Noorden 2009).

NRF2: AN ESSENTIAL COMPONENT FOR NADPH PRODUCTION, ALONG WITH CONTROLLING MANY OTHER PROCESSES

WHAT IS NRF2?

Our bodies have some really cool abilities to keep checks and balances. Nrf2 is one of my favorites.

Also known as nuclear factor (erythroid-derived 2)-like 2 and made by the NFE2L2 gene, Nrf2 is a transcription factor (a protein that helps specific genes turn on or off by binding to nearby DNA) that regulates various antioxidant enzymes and stress-response genes. Pronounced "nerf 2," the Nrf2 pathway is turned on when the body needs to make its own antioxidants. Present in every cell in the body, Nrf2 sends information to the cell's DNA, which consists of about 23,000 genes. Similar to the water in a building's sprinkler system, Nrf2 is stored away in the cell until it is needed to combat oxidative stress (put out a fire), when it is then released by the KEAP1 enzyme (kelch-like ECH-associated protein 1) into the nucleus. Think of KEAP1 as the sprinkler system and Nrf2 as the water.

KEAP1, which is produced by the KEAP1 gene, functions as a sensor for oxidants and electrophilic xenobiotics (Takaya et al. 2012) that damage the cell and disrupt metabolic processes. In addition to modulating the release of Nrf2, KEAP1 regulates the production of antioxidants like catalase and SOD (defined in Chapter 2), as well as detoxification enzymes, including glutathione S-transferase. While there are numerous factors and genes relating to SOD activity, I think now is a good time to mention that lower levels of SOD activity are associated with unsuccessful IVF outcomes (Tatone et al. 2015).

When Nrf2 is activated, it turns on hundreds of the "survival genes" in each cell's DNA while calming pro-inflammatory gene expression (Vomund 2017). It also activates detoxification and antioxidant defense and DNA repair, stabilizes proteins, and strengthens cellular integrity.

NERD NOTE FOR MY NERDIES: GENETIC VARIANTS AND AUTOPHAGY

I talked about mTOR and introduced autophagy in Chapter 4. Here is more detailed info on autophagy, the flip side of mTOR. If there are variants in any of these genes, pathway function may be more prone to compromise, eliciting a greater need for support.

NFE2L2 – also called the Nrf2 gene – modulates autophagy gene expression and regulates the expression of antioxidants in response to free radical production due to injury or inflammation. In addition to the critical functions of regulating antioxidant expression and modulating autophagy, Nrf2 also regulates iron sequestration, NADPH production, and the enzymes that reduce hydrogen peroxide. With all the critical functions that NADPH is used for, it is even more important to state that Nrf2 regulates NADPH production. It is truly the "head honcho in charge."

A great way to regulate Nrf2 activity is with molecular hydrogen tablets. Since Nrf2 acts like a sprinkler system and only turns on when needed, H2 causes Nrf2 to be expressed as needed and retained when not. While a sprinkler system can be lifesaving, we don't want it on all the time.

KEAP1 represses Nrf2 activation and releases it when inflammation comes along. Depending on which KEAP1 SNPs you have (differentiated by reference sequence number, more commonly referred to as "rs number" or "reference SNP"), KEAP1 variants can either inhibit Nrf2 release or make it too easily released, or "trigger happy." Also, Nrf2 and KEAP1 move us from mTOR to autophagy, so they impact cellular cleanup. Variants are cumulative, so the more variants you have, the worse off you may be, especially when those variants are homozygous.

ULK1 and ULK2: Initiation of autophagy requires ULK activity. If you have variants in KEAP1 and/or Nrf2-related genes, along with ULK1 and ULK2, you may have a much harder time moving into autophagy. Turmeric and resveratrol support Nrf2 by slowing mTOR while berberine and lithium support ULKs.

AMPK (AMP-activated protein kinase) is a key energy sensor and regulates cellular metabolism to maintain energy homeostasis (Kim et al. 2011). AMPK activates ULK1, a key initiator of autophagy. AMPK is also involved in mitochondrial function and blood sugar metabolism, both of which are essential to maintaining a pregnancy.

NRF2, NADPH, AND FOLATE

NADPH is needed for folate utilization and to help recycle homocysteine. Remember that elevated homocysteine stimulates NOX, which steals our NADPH so we can't use folate, and what a nasty cycle we can get our biochemical selves into.

Many people think they have a folate problem because of an MTHFR problem (Chapter 4 discusses why this is not likely the primary reason for a folate insufficiency), when it could instead be because of an NADPH problem that's due to an Nrf2 problem.

As I stated earlier in this chapter, NADPH is needed for glutathione recycling. Nrf2 also regulates glutathione production and expression. Without functional Nrf2, it doesn't matter how much glutathione you have in the body because it will not be usable.

Given how critical NAD+, NADPH, and NOX are in modulating oxidative stress, it is not surprising how important they are for both male and female fertility (notably endometriosis) (Nassif et al. 2016) and, in a broader picture, the pathobiology of many chronic human diseases.

NAD+ GOVERNS MATING ABILITY VIA THE SIRT GENES

Let's talk about the SIRT genes and how critical they are for mating ability. The family of SIRT genes, which stands for silent mating-type information regulation 2 proteins, are dependent on NAD+. Sirtuins are epigenetic regulators that control mating ability and DNA repair. They are involved in a wide array of physiological and pathological responses, such as stress resistance and inflammation, as well as regulating mitochondrial biogenesis and circadian clocks (Matsushima and Sadoshima 2015). A sirtuin's job is to sense biological stress in the environment, whether it's DNA damage, a change in temperature, or a lack of nutrients. Their job is to make an organism survive, which includes halting mating ability in order to repair damaged DNA because if we don't have healthy DNA, our offspring won't survive or thrive anyway.

Sirtuins control which genes to turn off and on in the face of adversity. They also talk to mTOR and other pathways related to longevity. And just like mTOR, sirtuins are also regulated by nutrients. This is especially true for NAD+, which declines as we age. Anything that increases NAD+ will increase SIRT1 activity.

As important as they are, sirtuins cannot function without NAD+. When NAD+ levels are high, sirtuins are more active. But at low NAD+ levels, sirtuin activities also decline, leading to aging. Since NAD+ is a rate-limiting factor for sirtuins, its modulation is emerging as a tool to regulate sirtuin function and oxidative metabolism.

Sirtuins are being recognized as one of the most integral factors in longevity and anti-aging, which affects fertility for sure.

The expression of sirtuins has been observed in mammalian ovaries, granulosa cells, oocytes, and embryos (Tatone et al. 2015).

SIRT1 inhibits mTOR (detailed in Chapter 4) and supports superoxide dismutase (SOD) activity and the vitamin D receptor (VDR) gene. Resveratrol is the most potent natural SIRT1 activator (Tatone et al. 2015). In direct regard to fertility, one study showed the stimulation of SIRT1 by resveratrol would be potentially beneficial in the treatment of luteal phase deficiency. These observations provide evidence for direct involvement of SIRT1 in upregulation of ovarian hormone secretion.

SIRT2 controls cell division and healthy egg production and is involved in chromosomal stability and longevity, DNA repair, cell cycle, apoptosis, metabolism, and aging (Donmez and Outeiro 2013).

SIRT3 provides support for the urea cycle and for the antioxidants superoxide dismutase (SOD genes) and catalase (CAT gene). SIRT3 stimulates AMPK for autophagy. It is considered critical for anti-aging and longevity. In regard to fertility, one study states, "Probably by acting as a sensor and regulator of ROS (free radicals called reactive oxygen species) levels and mitochondrial functions, SIRT3 has been recently found to exert a positive role in the folliculogenesis and luteinization processes in granulosa cells" (Tatone et al. 2015). SIRT3 also appears crucial in protecting early embryos against stress conditions (Tatone et al. 2018). Resveratrol and supporting NAD+ help stimulate SIRT3.

It's not just one SIRT that's important; it's the whole family of them, of which there are seven in mammals.

Anything that has to do with longevity and anti-aging will benefit fertility. Knowing which genes are key players in anti-aging and longevity and what SNPs they contain may give us an understanding of what support may be needed that was not addressed in previous protocols or treatments.

REFERENCES

Alleman, Rick J., Lalage A. Katunga, Margaret A. M. Nelson, David A. Brown, and Ethan J. Anderson. 2014. "The "Goldilocks Zone" from a redox perspective – Adaptive vs. deleterious responses to oxidative stress in striated muscle." *Frontiers in Physiology* 5, 358.

American Chemical Society. 2005. Nitric oxide could extend fertility. www.sciencedaily. com/releases/2005/09/050908084148.htm.

Becker, Y., U. Olshevsky, and Julia Levitt. 1967. "The role of arginine in the replication of herpes simplex virus." *Journal of General Virology* 1, no. 4, 471–478.

Bertoldo, Michael J., Dave R. Listijono, Wing-Hong Jonathan Ho, Angelique H. Riepsamen, Dale M. Goss, Dulama Richani, Xing L. Jin, et al. 2020. "NAD+ repletion rescues female fertility during reproductive aging." *Cell Reports* 30, no. 6, 1670–1681.

Blum, Kenneth, Marlene Oscar-Berman, Elizabeth Stuller, David Miller, John Giordano, Siobhan Morse, Lee McCormick, et al. 2012. "Neurogenetics and nutrigenomics of neuro-nutrient therapy for reward deficiency syndrome (RDS): clinical ramifications as a function of molecular neurobiological mechanisms." *Journal of Addiction Research & Therapy* 3, no. 5, 139.

Donmez, Gizem, and Tiago F. Outeiro. 2013. "SIRT1 and SIRT2: emerging targets in neuro-degeneration." *EMBO Molecular Medicine* 5, no. 3, 344–352.

Eid, Assaad A., Bridget M. Ford, Basant Bhandary, Rita de Cassia Cavaglieri, Karen Block, Jeffrey L. Barnes, Yves Gorin, Goutam Ghosh Choudhury, and Hanna E. Abboud. 2013. "Mammalian target of rapamycin regulates Nox4-mediated podocyte depletion in diabetic renal injury." *Diabetes* 62, no. 8, 2935–2947.

Fessel, Joshua P., and William M. Oldham. 2018. "Pyridine dinucleotides from molecules to man." *Antioxidants & Redox Signaling* 28, no. 3, 180–212.

Guemez-Gamboa, Alicia, Ana María Estrada-Sánchez, Teresa Montiel, Blanca Páramo, Lourdes Massieu, and Julio Morán. 2011. "Activation of NOX2 by the stimulation of ionotropic and metabotropic glutamate receptors contributes to glutamate neurotoxicity in vivo through the production of reactive oxygen species and calpain activation." *Journal of Neuropathology & Experimental Neurology* 70, no. 11, 1020–1035.

Imai, Shin-ichiro, and Leonard Guarente. 2014. "NAD+ and sirtuins in aging and disease." *Trends in Cell Biology* 24, no. 8, 464–471.

Kim, Joungmok, Mondira Kundu, Benoit Viollet, and Kun-Liang Guan. 2011. "AMPK and mTOR regulate autophagy through direct phosphorylation of Ulk1." *Nature Cell Biology* 13, no. 2, 132–141.

Krzastek, Sarah C., Jack Farhi, Marisa Gray, and Ryan P. Smith. 2020. "Impact of environmental toxin exposure on male fertility potential." *Translational Andrology and Urology* 9, no. 6, 2797.

Liwa, A. C., E. N. Barton, W. C. Cole, and C. R. Nwokocha. 2017. "Bioactive plant molecules, sources and mechanism of action in the treatment of cardiovascular disease." In *Pharmacognosy Fundamentals, Applications and Strategies*, 315–336. Academic Press.

Máté, Gábor, Lori R. Bernstein, and Attila L. Török. 2018. "Endometriosis is a cause of infertility. Does reactive oxygen damage to gametes and embryos play a key role in the pathogenesis of infertility caused by endometriosis?" *Frontiers in Endocrinology* 9, 725.

Matsushima, Shouji, and Junichi Sadoshima. 2015. "The role of sirtuins in cardiac disease." *American Journal of Physiology-Heart and Circulatory Physiology* 309, no. 9, H1375–H1389.

Mörlin, B., E. Andersson, B. Byström, and M. Hammarström. 2005. "Nitric oxide induces endometrial secretion at implantation time." *Acta Obstetricia et Gynecologica Scandinavica* 84, no. 11, 1029.

Nassif, J., S. A. Abbasi, A. Nassar, A. Abu-Musa, and A. A. Eid. 2016. "The role of NADPH-derived reactive oxygen species production in the pathogenesis of endometriosis: a novel mechanistic approach." *Journal of Biological Regulators and Homeostatic Agents* 30, no. 1, 31–40.

National Institutes of Health. n.d. Niacin fact sheet for health professionals. https://ods.od.nih.gov/factsheets/Niacin-HealthProfessional/.

National Library of Medicine. n.d. MTR gene. https://medlineplus.gov/genetics/gene/mtr/#conditions.

Peters, Anna L., and Cornelis J. F. Van Noorden. 2009. "Glucose-6-phosphate dehydrogenase deficiency and malaria: cytochemical detection of heterozygous G6PD deficiency in women." *Journal of Histochemistry & Cytochemistry* 57, no. 11, 1003–1011.

Pizzorno, Joseph. 2014. "Homocysteine: friend or foe?" *Integrative Medicine: A Clinician's Journal* 13, no. 4, 8.

Smith, Sheryl S., Barry D. Waterhouse, John K. Chapin, and Donald J. Woodward. 1987. "Progesterone alters GABA and glutamate responsiveness: a possible mechanism for its anxiolytic action." *Brain Research* 400, no. 2, 353–359.

Takaya, Kai, Takafumi Suzuki, Hozumi Motohashi, Ko Onodera, Susumu Satomi, Thomas W. Kensler, and Masayuki Yamamoto. 2012. "Validation of the multiple sensor mechanism of the Keap1-Nrf2 system." *Free Radical Biology and Medicine* 53, no. 4, 817–827.

Tatone, Carla, Giovanna Di Emidio, Arcangelo Barbonetti, Gaspare Carta, Alberto M. Luciano, Stefano Falone, and Fernanda Amicarelli. 2018. "Sirtuins in gamete biology and reproductive physiology: emerging roles and therapeutic potential in female and male infertility." *Human Reproduction Update* 24, no. 3, 267–289.

Tatone, Carla, Giovanna Di Emidio, Maurizio Vitti, Michela Di Carlo, Silvano Santini, Anna Maria D'Alessandro, Stefano Falone, and Fernanda Amicarelli. 2015. "Sirtuin functions in female fertility: possible role in oxidative stress and aging." *Oxidative Medicine and Cellular Longevity* 2015.

Vomund, Sandra, Anne Schäfer, Michael J. Parnham, Bernhard Brüne, and Andreas Von Knethen. 2017. "Nrf2, the master regulator of anti-oxidative responses." *International Journal of Molecular Sciences* 18, no. 12, 2772.

Woodbury, Anna, Shan Ping Yu, Ling Wei, and Paul García. 2013. "Neuro-modulating effects of honokiol: a review." *Frontiers in Neurology* 4, 130.

Zhang, Lili, Xiaoyan Wang, Yan Wu, Xiangru Lu, Peter Chidiac, Guoping Wang, and Qingping Feng. 2018. "Maternal diabetes up-regulates NOX2 and enhances myocardial ischaemia/reperfusion injury in adult offspring." *Journal of Cellular and Molecular Medicine* 22, no. 4, 2200–2209.

Appendix 13

APPENDIX 13A: PHASE 1 AND 2 LIVER DETOXIFICATION

Phase 1 liver detoxification involves the cytochrome P450 (CYP) genes. There are many different CYP genes involved with detoxifying a vast array of substances, both exogenous and endogenously produced. As I stated in Chapter 13, phase 1 liver detoxification takes these toxins or substances and transforms them into reactive intermediates with the help of the cytochrome P450 mono-oxygenase (CYP) enzymes, which are made by an array of CYP genes. These intermediary metabolites are often more toxic than the original toxin, so we want to ensure that phase 2 liver detoxification is supported and working effectively.

Clinical pearl: CYP enzymes are NADPH dependent, so if there are issues with NADPH or Nrf2 (discussed in Appendix 11), then there can be CYP/phase 1 detox issues, regardless of your CYP genetic profile.

In phase 2, which is heavily nutrient dependent, these intermediates are bound to substances (like sulfur groups, methyl groups, and acetyl groups) that help them turn water soluble so they can easily be excreted in the feces (via bile) and urine. There are six phase 2 liver detoxification pathways, and I discuss five of them in this book. I believe these pathways must be examined when someone is having health or fertility challenges. They are methylation (detailed in Chapter 4), sulfonation, glucuronidation, glutathione conjugation, and acetylation.

APPENDIX 13B: SULFATION/SULFONATION

For folks who have recently gotten MTHFR on their radar, CBS is typically the next gene they learn about. The CBS gene codes for the enzyme cystathionine-beta-synthase, which is the first step in the transsulfuration pathway that metabolizes sulfur-containing amino acids and is responsible for converting homocysteine into cysteine, which is the rate-limiting factor for glutathione production.

Some people, especially in MTHFR forums, say they can't tolerate sulfur-rich foods because of a CBS mutation. That's not typically what is happening though. It may be a sulfite-to-sulfate conversion issue due to variants in the SUOX gene or insufficient conversion cofactors like molybdenum. It could be an issue with excess oxalates, as mentioned in Chapter 9, because oxalates and sulfate compete for cellular transporters and receptors. Due to the fact that oxalates can hitch a ride everywhere that sulfur needs to be, they can get into the tissues in almost any part of the body.

Sulfites occur via the process of fermentation and can be found naturally in a number of foods and beverages. Our bodies also make sulfite when we process sulfur-containing amino acids.

If someone's body is overwhelmed by oxalates, adding sulfur can cause them to be dumped into the blood and elicit unpleasant symptoms.

If sulfates (like Epsom salts or chondroitin) cause a pain response, it may be due to an oxalate issue because the sulfate is causing oxalates to be displaced from tissues. If you get brain fog or a general feeling of toxicity from sulfites (people that experience this after only a few sips of wine), it may be more of an issue being able to convert sulfite to sulfate. Other symptoms of conversion issues are a skin response like hives, as well as abdominal pain and diarrhea.

In addition to being the main pathway for the metabolism of estrogens, sulfation/ sulfonation is an important phase 2 liver detox pathway for:

- Toxins
- Neurotransmitters
- Drugs
- Food dyes
- Bile acids
- Lipids
- Heavy metals
- Xenobiotic compounds
- Thyroid hormones
- Retinol
- Vitamin D

The family of SULT enzymes made by the sulfotransferase (SULT) (meaning to transfer sulfur groups from one place to another) genes make sulfation happen by converting these substances into less reactive, water-soluble substances by adding sulfur groups to them.

The sulfur group that the SULT enzymes transfer is derived from the PAPS enzyme, which is the universal sulfate donor and is coded for by the PAPS gene. Every single SULT enzyme uses PAPS as a cofactor. Variants on the PAPS genes can reduce sulfonation capacity and be very detrimental in allowing the body to break down and clear these compounds, which are usually very water soluble and readily excreted in the urine. Many of the toxins that we are exposed to on a daily basis block the sulfonation pathway: PCBs, BPA, and potentially other bisphenols and triclosan, to name a few.

There are five SULT families, each targeting a different set of substrates (molecules or substances that are acted upon by enzymes) and expressed in tissues throughout the body.

The SULT genes with plenty of research relating to hormones are SULT1 and SULT2.

SULT1 isoforms have been identified in the fetal brain, and it is clear that significant alterations in sulfotransferase activity take place during development, suggesting that sulfotransferases play a critical role in the development of the central nervous system (Hartzell and Seneff 2012). Also, some SULTs may play a role in detox processes occurring in the developing human fetus (Jančová and Šiller 2012).

SULT1, which includes five subtypes, is the best known of the sulfotransferase families. A few noteworthy SULTs relating directly to fertility are:

- SULT1A1 are involved with estrone and estrogen receptors.
- SULT1Bs target thyroid hormones.
- SULT1Cs target xenobiotics.
- SULT1Es target estrogenic steroids.

SULT2 enzymes are involved with sulfonating cholesterol and other hydroxysteroids such as pregnenolone, DHEA, and other neurosteroids.

APPENDIX 13C: SUOX

Sulfites turn into sulfates via the SUOX enzyme (from the SUOX gene). Genetic variants in the SUOX gene or inadequate levels of the primary cofactor molybdenum will result in SUOX enzyme activity weakness, which can result in less-than-optimal sulfate levels for phase 2 sulfation.

The SUOX enzyme is temperamental. It can be damaged through the depletion of molybdenum and overwhelmed by too many sulfite-containing foods, from tungsten poisoning, and through damage to folate metabolism.

Clinical pearl: The heme pathway is disrupted by glyphosate, which is the stated active ingredient in RoundUp. The SUOX enzyme is dependent on heme; therefore, glyphosate can disrupt your body's ability to convert sulfite to sulfate and allow for all kinds of problems associated with low sulfate, like oxalate issues and hormone imbalances. Go organic!

A methylation plasma profile from Doctor's Data or Genova Diagnostics can allow you to see how well the transsulfuration pathway is working and where wrenches in the system might be. You can then test sulfates and sulfites in urine with test strips that you can buy at a pharmacy. Having this information, coupled with the genetics and blood testing, you can see what's going on and if genetic variants are being expressed.

Regarding the urine test strips, if someone's urine sulfites are zero but sulfates are low at 200 (should be about 800), nothing is moving down the transsulfuration pathway. This can be an indication of not detoxing well because of blocks farther up, possibly because of genetics or low B6 status.

If someone presents with low sulfite and very high (1,600) sulfate levels, that is sulfate wasting, a great indicator of elevated oxalates because of the gradient that's created. Oxalates will force sulfates into the urine, and you will see it in urine at high levels. You may also see elevations if someone is doing a lot of high sulfates with things like Epsom, MSM, glucosamine, or chondroitin. If someone is doing all these things and urinary sulfate is not high, this can also indicate an oxalate issue.

Remember earlier in the book when I made it loud and clear that enzymes can't work without nutritional cofactors? Here's another perfect example. A nutritional cofactor insufficiency can inhibit enzymatic functioning even if there are no genetic variants in SUOX, CBS, or SULT genes. It is also important to note that our bodies do NOT have an inexhaustible ability to make enzymes. Stated differently, we can exhaust our enzyme potential, also referred to as our "enzyme reserve." This enzyme deficiency can be expedited by a nutrient-deficient, high-calorie diet of cooked (enzyme devoid) and/or processed foods, excess stress (from any source), the strain of extreme physical demands, and even genetic predispositions, etc. This forces the body once again to "rob Peter to pay Paul" by stealing enzymes from other storage depots so the pancreas can convert them to digestive enzymes in an effort to effectively and efficiently support the first and most important step of metabolism: digestion. This is why it is important to eat at least some of your organic produce raw and not to overcook other foods.

If SULT genes are not working for some reason, it is possible that sulfite is high and not being used for sulfation. Molybdenum is a primary cofactor for the enzymatic conversion of sulfite into sulfate, assisting SUOX gene activity. Even if the SULT gene isn't variated, if it doesn't have molybdenum, you may not have that conversion. This can cause excess sulfites and insufficient sulfation and transsulfuration.

Oxalates aside, people with variants in the SULT gene are more predisposed to having impaired detox ability and may be sensitive to toxins, heavy metals, and xenobiotics.

APPENDIX 13D: FOR MOST MAMMALIAN SPECIES, XENOBIOTIC BIOTRANSFORMATION[1] HAPPENS VIA THE GLUCURONIDATION PATHWAY

The UGT genes play a major part in this pathway. They do this by taking a toxin (which is typically fat soluble) and binding it to glucuronic acid (a type of sugar) to make it water soluble so that it can be excreted in the urine and feces via bile conjugation. There are many UGT genes, each having an affinity for certain substances. For instance, UGT2B15 serves as a major detoxification pathway of BPA, while bilirubin is exclusively metabolized by UGT1A1, and opioids by UGT2B7.

Glucuronidation is also necessary for the breakdown of fat-soluble vitamins (A, D, E, K), fatty acids, bile, serotonin, and melatonin. If someone has reduced glucuronidation, either from poor gut or liver health or genetic polymorphisms in UGT genes, or if the pathway is just completely inundated/overwhelmed, they likely will have problems detoxifying these compounds, potentially leading to negative downstream effects.

Gut dysbiosis may reduce and even reverse glucuronidation ability. Beta-glucuronidase is an enzyme produced by a subset of bacteria in a dysbiotic gut, including E. coli. This enzyme allows for the recirculation of the toxic compounds, even if there are no genetic variants in UGT genes, and the liver pathway is fine. High levels of beta-glucuronidase can lead to estrogen dominance because it causes estrogen to recirculate. The DUTCH test is a great way to see what is functionally happening with glucuronidation. Refer back to Chapter 13 for common inhibitors of glucuronidation.

APPENDIX 13E: CYSTEINE

Cysteine is made from cystathionine via the CTH gene in the transsulfuration pathway, for which pyridoxal phosphate (P5P – my favorite form of vitamin B6) is a cofactor. The genes/enzymes GCLM and GCLC then take glutamic acid/glutamate and cysteine and combine them with glycine, which is made with the help of the SHMT gene. The glutathione synthetase gene (GSS) then works its magic to assemble the antioxidant glutathione, but it can only do this with the help of ATP.

Many practitioners reach for N-acetyl-cysteine (NAC) to boost glutathione in their clients/patients. Variants in GCLM, GCLC, and GSS will significantly impact glutathione levels, and supplementing with NAC won't help compensate because it's not that there's a lack of cysteine (unless there are CTH variants or B6 deficiency); it's a lack of an enzyme to assemble the glutathione molecule, once cysteine is present.

GST is the primary phase 2 enzyme that turns glutathione into a detoxifying agent as opposed to an antioxidant. The GST enzyme in glutathione conjugation is used for clearing toxins like acrylonitrile, ethylene oxide, xylene, benzene, 1,3-butadiene, propylene, 1-bromopropane, and a couple types of mycotoxins, to name a few.

When it comes to detoxifying mycotoxins, almost every practitioner will include glutathione. This can be useless for mycotoxin detox, unless those mycotoxins are ochratoxin-A and aflatoxin B-1, which are most commonly caused by water damage. As far as research shows, glutathione conjugation, via the GST genes, only clears those two. In comparison, glucuronidation clears at least eleven, a few of which have studies associating them with various reproductive/fertility issues. While glucuronidation is not the primary clearance pathway for ochratoxin and aflatoxin B-1, it will pick up the slack when glutathione conjugation is insufficient.

Mycotoxins decrease the formation of glutathione production by changing gene expression (GCL genes). So even if you don't have any GCLC or GCLM variants, mycotoxins can still mimic a polymorphism.

Ochratoxin inhibits Nrf2, which is needed for the expression of GCLM, GCLC, GSTs, and GSS (glutathione synthetase, which assembles the three amino acids to make the antioxidant glutathione). It is also needed for NADPH production and expression in order to reduce glutathione. Basically, ochratoxin is able to inhibit its own detoxification. What this means is that with ochratoxin's capacity to inhibit Nrf2, it doesn't matter how much glutathione you have in the body or how well your GSTs are working; they are unable to perform and detox.

APPENDIX 13F: THE ACETYL COENZYME-A ACETYLTRANSFERASE (ACAT) ENZYME

The acetyl coenzyme-A acetyltransferase (ACAT) enzyme, made by ACAT gene, is what converts dietary fats and proteins into acetyl-CoA, which makes ATP. Pantethine, an active derivative of vitamin B5, is required for this conversion process. Someone with ACAT variants or B5 insufficiency may have issues making acetyl-CoA and, therefore, may have ATP issues. And remember, if the body is not producing energy efficiently, it will know it is not an optimal time to create a baby (Figure 1 Appendix 13F).

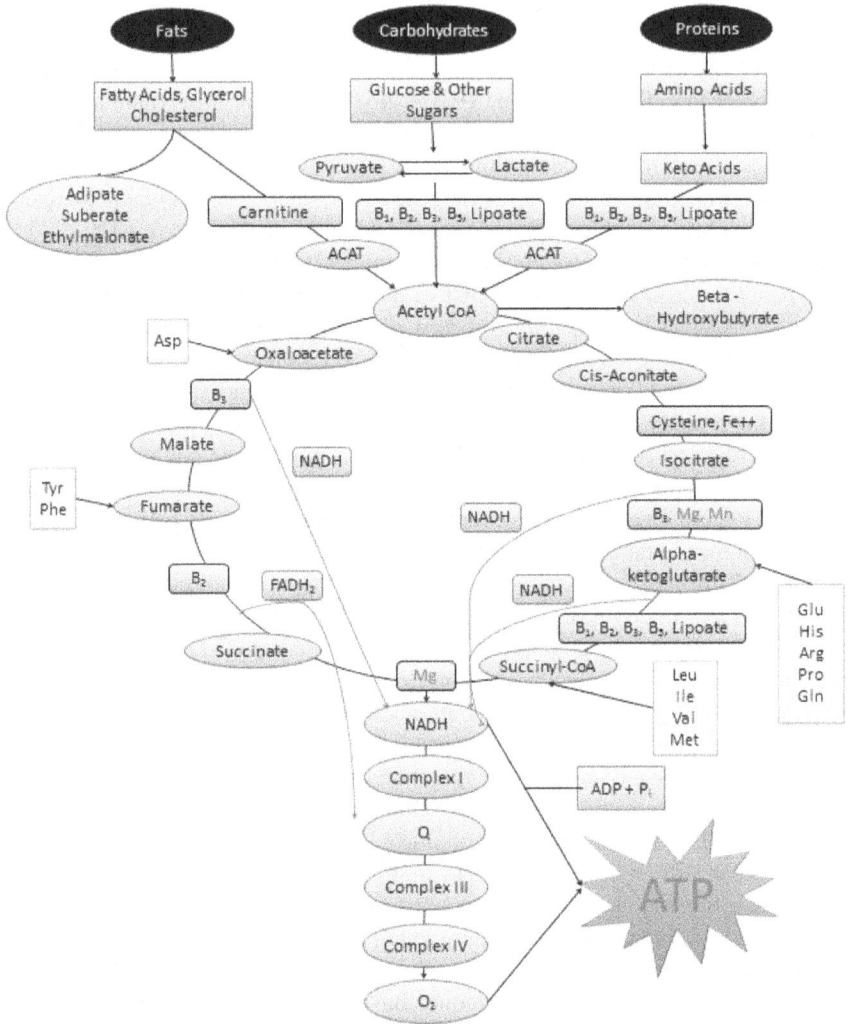

FIGURE 1 APPENDIX 13F   The ACAT gene is what converts dietary fats and proteins into acetyl CoA, which ultimately makes ATP.

Source: Courtesy of NutriGenetic Research Institute

The proper use of pantethine/vitamin B5 depends on the pantothenate kinase (PANK) enzyme, made by the PANK gene. Variants in PANK genes may have a negative impact on the utilization of B5 and hinder the production of acetyl-CoA. PANK participates in the first step in the creation of CoA. Because CoA is a ubiquitous and essential cofactor in all organisms (they all need to produce energy!), the PANK genes that make up this pathway are essential for all organism survival and growth (Yang et al. 2006). Because of this, PANK variants may be more impactful than MTHFR variants.

Pantethine is highly water soluble. If the body isn't using it, it will be excreted, so it is not concerning if this marker (pantothenic/B5) is elevated on a urine organic acids test. When supplementing with pantethine, taking smaller doses throughout the day is better than one larger dose, in my opinion.

PHASE II DETOXIFICATION CONJUGATION BY ACETYLATION

The N-acetyltransferase enzymes, coded for by the NAT1 and NAT2 genes, are involved in the metabolism of a wide array of different substances that we are exposed to on a daily basis. The NAT genes are what take the acetyl group from acetyl-CoA and transfer it to the toxin or chemical compound in the detox process of acetylation. Adequate acetyl-CoA and NAT gene function is needed for proper acetylation. The NAT genes also help clear systemic mold, fungus, and yeast. I talk more about mold and mycotoxins in Chapter 7.

As I stated, phase 2 acetylation is involved in eliminating xenobiotics, histamine, serotonin, and sulfa drugs. If someone is sensitive to chemicals like car exhaust or cigarette smoke, or they get drunk very easily, they may be a "slow" acetylator, which may be caused by genetic predisposition in PANK, ACAT, and/or NAT genes. Smokers, second-hand smoke, eating charred foods, and air pollution will fill someone's "acetylation bucket" faster.

PANK IS NEEDED FOR HEALTHY FATS, WHICH MAKE HORMONES

PANK activity is needed to make ACAT reactions that create acetyl-CoA for lipid synthesis. Proper lipid synthesis is needed for the steroidal pathway, which makes sex and stress hormones, to function properly, with emphasis being on cortisol, which knocks down histamine and inflammation. This helps keep hormones balanced.

If we are low in cortisol production due to PANK or ACAT variants (among various other possible reasons), the body will steal energy from digestion and elimination to try to keep up with the cortisol demand. We will see a big swing in hormones, especially depletion of progesterone.

One of progesterone's many functions is to suppress mast cell activation. If we have low progesterone from PANK or ACAT variants or from low cortisol, we can become vulnerable to mast cell activation.

Here's a typical scenario: Acetylation clears histamine. If there are acetylation issues, excess histamine will stimulate mast cells and NOX activity (described in Chapter 11). But NOX also stimulates mast cell activity, which creates more histamine. You can see how this is a vicious cycle.

In direct relation to fertility, one study states that the acetylation status of proteins in oocytes is positively or negatively associated with oocyte aging (Tatone et al. 2015).

This all comes back to the central premise of this book that if we have issues with energy production and inflammation, the body will sure as heck know there is not enough energy to grow a baby.

NOTE

1   The chemical transformation of a toxin into a water-soluble compound that can be excreted.

REFERENCES

Hartzell, Samantha, and Stephanie Seneff. 2012. "Impaired sulfate metabolism and epi-
    genetics: is there a link in autism?" *Entropy* 14, no. 10, 1953–1977.
Jančová, Petra, and Michal Šiller. 2012. "Phase II drug metabolism." *Topics on Drug
    Metabolism* 35–60.
Tatone, Carla, Giovanna Di Emidio, Maurizio Vitti, Michela Di Carlo, Silvano Santini, Anna
    Maria D'Alessandro, Stefano Falone, and Fernanda Amicarelli. 2015. "Sirtuin func-
    tions in female fertility: possible role in oxidative stress and aging." *Oxidative Medicine
    and Cellular Longevity* 2015.
Yang, Kun, Yvonne Eyobo, Leisl A. Brand, Dariusz Martynowski, Diana Tomchick, Erick
    Strauss, and Hong Zhang. 2006. "Crystal structure of a type III pantothenate kinase:
    insight into the mechanism of an essential coenzyme A biosynthetic enzyme univer-
    sally distributed in bacteria." *Journal of Bacteriology* 188, no. 15, 5532–5540.

Appendix 15

Many enzymes along the histamine pathway are copper dependent. Superoxide dismutase (SOD), made by the SOD gene, is one of them. SOD is an antioxidant made by the body, and its production is dependent on a healthy balance between copper and zinc. SOD neutralizes superoxide (SO). I discussed SOD in Appendix 2A.

I mention SOD here because elevated histamine increases NADPH-oxidase, or NOX, made by the NOX gene. NOX is discussed in Appendix 11A. Elevated NOX increases superoxide (SO) levels, which then uses up SOD, which triggers mast cells to release more histamine, leaving us more vulnerable to mast cell activation.

Someone can have no SNPs in SOD or copper-related genes (ceruloplasmin [CP] gene and SLC31A1 and SLC31A2, which are involved with copper absorption and transport), but like many people did during the pandemic of 2020, supplementing with high levels of zinc for prolonged periods of time can throw off the copper/zinc ratio. It's good to measure copper, zinc, and ceruloplasmin periodically to get an idea of what levels are and adjust accordingly.

Glossary of Terms

Allele – One of two versions of DNA sequence at any particular location. Alleles control characteristics and different alleles result in different genetic characteristics. People inherit two alleles, one from each parent. If the two alleles are the same, that person is homozygous for that allele. If the alleles are different, the individual is homozygous.

Antioxidant – A substance (either external or made by the body) that inhibits or neutralizes the oxidation effects of free radicals. Antioxidants work by donating electrons.

ATP – Abbreviation for adenosine 5′-triphosphate. ATP is present in all cells, where it is used to transport and store energy needed for biochemical reactions. ATP can be formed either in the general cytoplasm during glycolysis or in the mitochondria via the Krebs cycle and the electron transport system if oxygen is present.

Autonomic nervous system – The part of the nervous system that regulates involuntary action, such as heart rate, respiration, and digestion. It is divided into the sympathetic nervous system (fight, freeze, or flight) and the parasympathetic nervous system (rest, digest, repair, reproduce).

Bioavailable – The state in which a substance can be readily used by the body after administration.

Biotoxins – Toxins produced by a living organism.

Cortisol – A steroid hormone produced by the adrenal cortex (outer portion of the adrenal gland) that regulates carbohydrate metabolism, maintains blood pressure, and is released in response to stressors.

Doula – A person (most often a woman) who provides emotional, physical, and informational support to a woman during labor and childbirth, as well as in the postpartum period.

Dysbiosis – An imbalance of beneficial bacteria, usually referring to (but not limited to) the gut.

Endogenous – Originating or produced within an organism, tissue, or cell.

Enzymes – Organic substances (proteins) composed of amino acids that trigger and regulate chemical reactions in the body.

Epigenetics – The study of how your diet, lifestyle, stressors, and environment can cause changes affecting the way your genes work. Epigenetic changes are reversible and do not change your DNA sequence.

Exogenous – Originating externally. Not produced by the body.

Free radical – Any atom or molecule that has one or more unpaired electrons and is therefore highly reactive, seeking to acquire electrons from other substances. Electrons like to be in pairs to be stable.

Functional genomics – As defined in the *Encyclopedia of Bioinformatics and Computational Biology* (2019), a branch that integrates molecular biology and cell biology studies and deals with the whole structure, function, and regulation of a gene (and the proteins it produces) in contrast to the gene-by-gene approach of classical molecular biology. In other words, how the genes within the genome interact and affect the others' functioning. Looking at how things affect the functioning of our genes and how things cause genes to interact with each other.

Genome– All the genetic information in an organism's chromosomes and mitochondria.

Genomics – The dynamic interactions between all our genes and how they influence biochemical pathway functioning and physiology.

Glutathione – A compound made up of three amino acids: glutamic acid, cysteine, and glycine. It is essential for neutralizing free radicals and for detoxification. Glutathione is known as the "master antioxidant" because it is able to recycle itself and other antioxidants.

Inflammation – A protective response to injury, irritation, toxicity, or infection caused by physical, chemical, or biologic agents. Inflammation is often characterized by pain, swelling, redness, heat, or loss of function.

Limbic system – Interconnected parts of the brain involved with emotion and behavior (especially those involved with survival, like fear), as well as motivation, long-term memory, olfaction, and various autonomic functions.

Metabolism – The chemical reactions that take place in cells and organisms to create energy and maintain life.

Methylation – The addition of a methyl group to a molecule. Methylation is critical in gene expression and may be passed from one generation to the next. Methylation is also one of the liver's phase 2 detoxification pathways.

Methylfolate – The bioavailable form of vitamin B9.

Microvilli – Tiny finger-like projections on the surface of cells that greatly increase the surface area so as to increase nutrient absorption ability.

Nutrigenomics – The study of how nutrients, toxins, and stressors affect the functioning and expression of our genes and biochemical pathways.

Organic acid – A chemical compounds excreted in the urine of mammals that is a product of metabolism.

Oxalate – An organic acid found in plants and also made by the body and certain types of mold and fungus. The oxalates bind to minerals, creating nano-size jagged crystals that can shred tissue and create inflammation. Oxalates keep the body from being able to use the minerals.

Oxidative stress – Caused by an imbalance between the production of free radicals and the ability to neutralize them, leading to cell and tissue damage.

SNP – Single nucleotide polymorphism. A single site in any DNA sequence for which the identity of the nucleotide differs among individuals, often associated with a physiological variation, such as response to a drug, and used as a genetic marker.

Resources

These resources are products that I personally use and recommend to my clients and friends. Because of this, I have created affiliate accounts with some of them, and I may make a small commission if you choose to purchase through my link which won't result in any additional costs for you. Some, like the sauna, include coupon codes for a special discount for readers of this book.

My website www.JaclynDowns.com.

https://jaclyndowns.com/shop has links to products I personally use and love that I may not have mentioned in this book.

https://us.fullscript.com/welcome/jdowns is my online dispensary where you can get access to a ton of professional-line supplements that must be ordered through a health professional.

Follow me on Instagram @FunctionalFertilitySolutions.

WATER FILTRATION:

- AquaTru countertop reverse osmosis water system – http://shrsl.com/1vfsk-2ffl-12yt4.
- Zero countertop water filtration dispenser – https://amzn.to/3JMVAIx. (This link is for the large glass one.)

PORTABLE SAUNA

- Therasage – Full-spectrum infrared sauna – www.therasage.com. (Use coupon code **JDOWNSBOOK** for a special offer for readers of this book of a 15% discount on any purchase.)

RED LIGHT THERAPY

- Thera Tri-Light Panel – Therasage (www.therasage.com) one that can be placed directly on the skin! Again, use coupon code **JDOWNSBOOK** for 15% off.
- Platinum LED – https://platinumled.myshopify.com/discount/JDOWNS?aff=410. (Use coupon code JDOWNS for a 5% discount.)

DRAINAGE DETOX KIT

- PEKANA Big Three Basic Detoxification & Drainage Kit – Bioresource makes this. You can call to order and give them my name (Jaclyn Downs) as your reference. This kit includes three remedies that have a regulating effect on the liver, kidneys, and lymphatic system and help with the mobilization and excretion of toxins. (800) 203–3775.

MOLD RESOURCES – TESTING, INSPECTION, REMEDIATION

- The International Society for Environmentally Acquired Illness (ISEAI) – https://iseai.org/find-a-professional/.
- Immunolytics – https://immunolytics.com/?wpam_id=16. Mold plates that can take samples of rooms, surfaces, and even your pets. Video guides and step-by-step instructions will walk you through the sampling process, understanding the results, and sending samples to their lab for expert analysis.

FUNCTIONAL LAB TESTING

- Great Plains Laboratory – www.greatplainslaboratory.com/. They offer the urine organic acid test, which I have mentioned numerous times throughout this book, as well as a host of other tests.
- Precision Analytical – https://dutchtest.com/. The lab that provides the DUTCH testing I mention in this book. I consider them to be the gold standard in hormone testing.
- Vibrant Wellness – www.vibrant-wellness.com/. They offer many different types of testing, and even though I didn't mention them directly in the book, I think they are a great company and wanted to include them here.

OTHER HELPFUL RESOURCES

- Castor oil packs, kits, and accessories – Queen of the Thrones makes castor oil packs that are easier and way less messy than the DIY setup that I previously had. https://shop.queenofthethrones.com/functionalfertilitysolutions
- DetoxMe – https://web.detoxmeapp.org/. An app you can download that helps you make choices to reduce your exposure to harmful chemicals where you live, work, and play. It makes doing this almost like a game!
- Environmental Working Group – www.ewg.org. They have many resources to offer, including the Skin Deep cosmetics database and Guide to Sunscreens. I recommend this website for people just starting out on a clean living journey.
- Pesticide Action Network– www.whatsonmyfood.org. Reported findings by the USDA's Pesticide Data Program. Lists dozens of foods and the pesticides that they were found to contain.
- Inaura.com – An interactive platform that helps you find resources to support your healing, growth, and self-discovery journey. It features high-quality education, world-class professional guides, classes, workshops, and much more – across the full spectrum of mental, emotional, and spiritual well-being.
- *The Garden of Fertility* by Katie Singer – https://amzn.to/3P4997f. You will not only learn how to chart your fertility signals to determine when you are fertile and when you are not but also gain a deeper connection to and understanding of your body and health.

Index

Note: *Italic* page references indicate figures and shaded text.